THERAPIST GUIDE FOR
MAINTAINING
CHANGE

For bulk purchases at reduced prices of *Maintaining Change: A Personal Relapse Prevention Manual*, please contact the Sage Special Sales Department nearest you.

SAGE Publications, Inc.
2455 Teller Road
Thousand Oaks, California 91320
E-mail: order@sagepub.com

SAGE Publications Ltd.
6 Bonhill Street
London EC2A 4PU
United Kingdom

SAGE Publications India Pvt. Ltd.
M-32 Market
Greater Kailash I
New Delhi 110 048 India

THERAPIST GUIDE FOR

MAINTAINING
CHANGE

Relapse Prevention for Adult Male
Perpetrators of Child Sexual Abuse

Hilary Eldridge

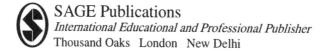

SAGE Publications
International Educational and Professional Publisher
Thousand Oaks   London   New Delhi

For information:

 SAGE Publications, Inc.
2455 Teller Road
Thousand Oaks, California 91320
E-mail: order@sagepub.com

SAGE Publications Ltd.
6 Bonhill Street
London EC2A 4PU
United Kingdom

SAGE Publications India Pvt. Ltd.
M-32 Market
Greater Kailash I
New Delhi 110 048 India

Printed in the United States of America

Library of Congress Cataloging-in-Publication Data

Eldridge, Hilary.
    Therapist Guide for Maintaining Change: Relapse Prevention for Adult
    Male Perpetrators of Child Sexual Abuse / by Hilary Eldridge.
        p.   cm.
    Includes bibliographical references and index.
    ISBN 0-7619-1130-8 (cloth: acid-free paper). —
        1. Child molesters—Rehabilitation.   2. Pedophilia—Relapse—
    Prevention.   3. Child sexual abuse—Prevention.   I. Title.
    RC560.C46E39   1997
    616.85'836—dc21   97-21154

This book is printed on acid-free paper.

98   99   00   01   02   03   10   9   8   7   6   5   4   3   2   1

Acquiring Editor:	C. Terry Hendrix
Editorial Assistant:	Dale Mary Grenfell
Production Editor:	Sherrise M. Purdum
Production Assistant:	Denise Santoyo
Typesetter/Designer:	Janelle LeMaster
Indexer:	Teri Greenberg
Cover Designer:	Candice Harman
Print Buyer:	Anna Chin

For *Lucy Faithfull*,
who spent her life campaigning for children
and believed that the best way to protect them
is to change offenders

Contents

Foreword

In the earlier version of this text Hilary Eldridge was kind enough to acknowledge the influence of some of my earlier work in the area of relapse prevention. Thus it seems appropriate that I return the favor by contributing a few prefatory comments to the commercial version of the manual.

When this manuscript was submitted to Sage Publications I was asked to review it. I recall saying that Hilary was not only a colleague but a personal friend, so I was prepared to like the text. What I was not prepared for, I said, was that I was going to like it as much as I did. I then went on to make some suggestions for improving the manuals, primarily by providing better linkage between the *Therapist Guide* and the *Perpetrator Manual*. These changes are reflected in the text you have before you.

My first knowledge of relapse prevention (RP) came to me in 1978. It was in the form of a manual given to me by Janice Marques, then a graduate student at the University of Washington, supervised by Alan Marlatt, the developer of the original model of RP. This was the alcohol/drug abuse version. She said, "I think there's something here that could be applied to sex offenders." Five years later the first paper by Pithers, Marques, Gibat, and Marlatt (1983) described the possible application to sex offenders. In the earlier version of *Maintaining Change* (1995) Bill Pithers quoted the late Fay Honey Knopp as saying that the introduction of relapse prevention was "a quiet revolution within the field." It may have been quiet at the start but it has been anything but quiet in the past 10 years. Karl Hanson (1996) has evaluated the professional and social impact of RP on the sex offender treatment field:

> the introduction of RP theory was highly motivating to sexual
> offender therapists. RP validated their perception that many sexual

offenders were at ongoing risk and, more importantly, explicitly defined the therapists' role as addressing these anticipated lapses. Instead of interpreting recidivism as evidence that sexual offenders were untreatable, RP viewed posttreatment behavioral deterioration as an expected and workable problem. (p. 203)

Hanson (1996) sums up his evaluation:

RP has provided direction and focus for a generation of sexual offender therapists. (p. 206)

That, I would submit, is no mean accomplishment.

Hilary Eldridge's *Maintaining Change* is directly in the mainstream of RP theory and practice and, to my mind, advances practice through its user friendliness. She states that the manuals may be introduced into existing programs. Here she is talking about the original RP model advanced by Marlatt and Gordon (1985) where the approach is used as a *maintenance program* following an existing cessation-oriented treatment program. In Hilary's scheme, treatment falls into three phases. Phase 1 has as its goal stimulating the client to recognize the need to change. Hilary's approach weaves RP into the treatment from the beginning although there is the flavor here of some of the more traditional approaches to sex offender treatment. Phase 2 is where RP strategies are introduced, the nuts and bolts of self-control and offense-free lifestyle maintenance. Phase 3 is the community follow-up portion using call-back sessions and the perpetrator's support network.

It is important to emphasize that RP was designed for people who want to change their behavior. Hilary notes that the *Maintaining Change* program is specifically designed for offenders who clearly show repetitive offense patterns. Not surprisingly, it uses a combination of traditional cognitive-behavioral approaches with the specific interventions characteristic of RP. It has been noted repeatedly in the literature that this is the combination that works best with sex offenders. In this interest I should mention that the 20 points expressed as the underlying philosophy of the program (pp. v-vi, this guide) represent an excellent list of requirements for development of a treatment program for sex offenders.

I mentioned earlier that these manuals are very user friendly. I should also state that this applies to both therapists and clients. We have used portions of *Maintaining Change* in our adult outpatient sex offender program with great success. The guidelines for therapists are clear and easy to implement. The information given to our clients, particularly homework assignments, is easy to understand and work with.

I believe that this is an excellent addition to the sex offender literature and I can personally endorse it and commend it to you. With materials like these, perhaps we can inspire a second generation of sex offender therapists.

—D. Richard Laws, Ph.D.
Victoria, British Columbia

Acknowledgments

The thrapist guide and the accompanying personal relapse prevention manual for perpetrators are based on principles described by D. Richard Laws, Ph.D., and William D. Pithers, Ph.D., in their work in the area of relapse prevention with sex offenders, and I would like to thank them both for their inspiration. I am especially grateful for the time Richard has taken to review this therapist guide at its different stages of development and to pilot the personal relapse prevention manual for perpetrators in his own program.

I am also indebted to Anna Salter, Ph.D., who persuaded me to publish these books, and to Barrie Bridgeman from the West Midlands Probation Service and Derek Perkins, Ph.D., from Broadmoor Hospital, who have given me their time, help, and support. I am grateful to everyone who contributed ideas to the project, to James McGuire, Ph.D., for his help regarding source material, and to David Thornton, Ph.D., who helped ensure that the manual can provide continuity between the British Prison Core Sex Offender Treatment Programme and community-based programs.

Many thanks go to the staff who piloted *Maintaining Change* in the STOP Programme at Peterhead Prison, in the West Midlands Probation Service's specialist unit, in the Somerset Probation Service, and in Broadmoor Hospital.

Special thanks are due to colleagues at the Gracewell Clinic and Lucy Faithfull Foundation, without whose cooperation and support *Maintaining Change* would not have been possible. I would also like to thank the offenders who were committed to an offense-free lifestyle, gave feedback on what worked for them, and contributed parts of their relapse prevention plans to help others avoid reoffending. The names used here have been changed in order to protect the identities of individual offenders, their victims, and families.

Part I

Using *Maintaining Change*

A Therapist Guide With Accompanying Manual for Perpetrators

The therapist guide is designed for use with *Maintaining Change: A Personal Relapse Prevention Manual.* The two books are presented in three matching phases, which are structured to provide material for use during the offender's progress through a therapy program. Together they form a cognitive behavioral module that can be integrated into the wider program.

The Therapist Guide

This guide provides a theoretical and practical base for using relapse prevention techniques. It includes information on patterns of offending, routes to relapse, and how to counter them. Guidelines and suggestions for integrating relapse prevention philosophy, exercises, and techniques into programs, draw on experience of piloting the manual in community-based, residential, secure hospital, and prison prgrams.

Three phases of intervention/therapy are described, corresponding with the three phases laid out in the personal relapse prevention manual, including the rationale for the exercises within each phase, ways of introducing and exploring them, and motivating offenders.[1]

1

The Personal Relapse Prevention Manual

This manual contains explanatory material written for offenders and presented in the form of handouts and exercises relating to the offending cycle/pattern, likely routes to relapse, and key thoughts, feelings, and behavioral patterns along these routes. They are designed and organized for use during the three phases of intervention/therapy described in this therapist's guide.

The emphasis is on the offender developing his own personalized relapse prevention plan, hence the standard materials can be modified by the offender and therapist working together. During the therapy/ maintenance process, the offender will find that certain exercises are particularly helpful to him, and he may generate a variety of ways of remembering or triggering into the ideas or feelings he experiences in using them. By the time he moves out of his therapy program, he may distill these into key phrases or devices that relate to thoughts, feelings, and actions that can help him cope with risky scenarios, moods, and lapses.

Rationale for the Work

For many years, work with perpetrators of child sexual abuse emphasized assessment and treatment, with only a minor focus on the need for offenders to learn strategies to maintain change in the long term. Increasingly, it is becoming accepted that for many offenders, maintaining change will be a lifelong occupation. A habit has been acquired that appears to be independent of the factors that predisposed its original development. Where the habit has become a maladaptive coping mechanism for dealing with situational and emotional problems, the habit itself requires attention if reoffending is to be prevented.

Although not all offenders have repetitive cycles or patterns, many do. Hence, it is important in assessment to look for the likelihood of one existing. If we don't entertain the possibility, the offender will certainly not enlighten us: most initially deny the existence of such patterns to professionals, and sometimes to themselves as well. Admission of a pattern is tantamount to admitting responsibility, something which many offenders find very painful.

Maintaining Change: A Personal Relapse Prevention Manual is designed for use with those offenders who have been assessed as having repetitive patterns, and have entered a therapy program, ideally one which combines individual and groupwork components.

Arguments continue about the advantages of one type of therapy over another, but in recent years, the use of a range of approaches in combination has been recognized to be most effective, a view supported by a study of treatment outcome (Marshall, Jones, Ward, Johnston, & Barbaree, 1991). Thoughts, feelings, and behaviors contribute to sex offending, and these need to be addressed in therapy. Therapy needs to focus on the attitudes and beliefs that legitimate offending for the perpetrator, and on the sexual arousal pattern that may have become conditioned around it. Behavioral techniques can be effective for controlling deviant sexual fantasies, but offenders have no reason to use them if they believe their offending has done no harm or that it was justified. Hence, these techniques are combined with psychotherapeutic and cognitive restructuring programs to address issues such as attitudes to women and children, power in relationships, unresolved feelings about childhood victim experiences, and current perception of self in relation to others.

Therapies that focus on the offender gaining insight into the causes of his behavior do not look so promising. According to Salter (1988), "This is because the development of insight has not been demonstrated, by itself, to decrease sexual acting out, even as it has not been shown to control other addictive behaviors" (p. 129). Field and Williams (1970) term the results of psychoanalytic treatment with sex offenders "disappointing"; and they found that their offenders questioned whether even if a psychoanalytic explanation "were understood and accepted, this knowledge alone would give to him sufficient control over his impulses to avoid the next offense" (p. 29). Given that there are so many variables affecting a person's development, it seems likely that a search for the reason why someone became a sex offender may in itself be a misguided mystery tour, often misled by the offender who may prefer to look for explanations rather than to prevent reoffending. Roger Wolfe, of North West Treatment Associates in Seattle, once commented that psychotherapy used alone simply produced "sex offenders with insight" (quoted in Salter, 1988, p. 130).

Salter (1988) comments that "compulsive behaviors respond first and foremost to cognitive/behavioral techniques." However, she points out that the use of such techniques does not mean that emotion or cognition are ignored in the push to change inappropriate sexual behavior. The emotional states that precede and that occur during the offense are carefully attended to as well as the cognitions that release the behavior at the time and justify it afterwards. Nor is it inappropriate at times to explore with an offender the origins of his need for power and control over children, or of his anger. (p. 130)

Marshall et al. (1991) describe improvements made to their own program that have had encouraging results:

From 1984 on, Marshall et al. increased the focus on relationship issues, particularly the need to accept the responsibilities entailed in relationships and to develop activities which enhance intimacy. The assertiveness component was intensified, and decreased emphasis was placed on the strictly sexual aspects of the behavior; a relapse prevention (internal management) component was also added. (p. 480)

The majority of habitual child sexual abuse perpetrators have behavior rather than mental health problems. Currently, most programs for offenders emphasize that it is inappropriate to talk in terms of cure, as if the offender has an illness. Instead, emphasis is placed on the offender learning to change his thinking and behavioral patterns and control his sexuality. However, the very term used most often to refer to this process, *treatment*, tends to belie this approach; it seems to suggest that the perpetrator will be "treated" and will then somehow be "better." Hence there is often a lack of emphasis on how the perpetrator will maintain change in the long term. This is a particularly difficult problem for long-established, habitual offenders.

It is important that both therapist and offender recognize that however much the offender learns about the harm he has done, and however strongly he begins to empathize with his victims, and however many techniques he learns to try to restructure his sexual arousal pattern, there will be times when he experiences a strong desire to reoffend. For many perpetrators, sexual abuse has become a key part of their social as well as sexual lives, and unless interventions are firmly anchored to relapse prevention, they are unlikely to be effective in the long term. An offender may make good progress during therapy, but may have difficulty maintaining an offense-free life unless he learns effective coping mechanisms and plans how to use them to deal with the likelihood that at some stage he may want to reoffend.

The therapist needs to emphasize the notion of *control* rather than cure in working with the offender. Perhaps some change in terminology is necessary in order to ensure that the therapist does not pay lip service to the notion of control while unwittingly colluding with the offender's tendency to avoid taking responsibility for his own behavior and for changing it. The belief that one can be treated by a professional who will effect a cure fits neatly with the tendency, common among sex abuse perpetrators, to place responsibility outside the self. *Treatment* may perhaps be more appropriately renamed *intervention* or *therapy*.

The ways in which relapse prevention concepts are applied in practice are somewhat variable (Marshall & Anderson, 1996). In this book, I outline components of a relapse prevention model, but I seek to encourage therapists to translate these into user-friendly language that perpetrators can relate to their own lives, rather than teach them how to sound like they just digested an academic tome. The accompanying personal relapse prevention manual is designed with the same goal in mind. To use a "Salterism," talking the technical talk is very different from talking about real-life experiences and walking the offense-free walk in the real world.

Underlying Principles for Use of *Maintaining Change: A Personal Relapse Prevention Manual*

It is assumed that an assessment of the offender has been completed prior to intervention. This assessment may have included the taking of personal and family histories as well as the use of offense- and personality-related measures such as those described by Beckett, Beech, Fisher, and Fordham (1994).

The personal relapse prevention manual is intended for use as part of a planned program of intervention under the guidance of a professionally qualified and experienced therapist who has access to appropriate training, supervision, and support. The program should include a regular review of both the progress of individual perpetrators and overall program effectiveness.

The personal relapse prevention manual is designed to be generally accessible, and the exercises contained in it are described there in some detail. However, some offenders may need additional help, and care should be taken to ensure that each offender clearly understands the tasks to be completed. Some of the exercises are variations on a theme, as it can help to focus on the same issue from different angles in order to develop a greater understanding. However, certain exercises may be used as alternatives to each other, if the therapist prefers.

A core principle of the personal relapse prevention manual and this therapist's guide is that relapse prevention should be an integral part of any program of intervention. The manual can be used in work with an individual or incorporated into a group work program. It will integrate particularly well with programs that address the thinking, feeling, and behavior patterns of offenders in relation to the following:

- Patterns or cycles of offending
- Cognitive distortions—general and situational
- Cognitive empathy
- Affect empathy
- Sexuality
- Social relationships
- Self

The operating principles of the intervention program should include the following:

- Professionals working with the offender take the view that they are, first and foremost, agents of child protection.
- In line with the above, the professionals adopt a policy of responsible information sharing with appropriate child protection agencies.
- Therapy takes place within a therapeutic environment.
- The offender is encouraged to take a positive and active approach to himself and his therapy, regardless of whether positive or aversive techniques are used in therapy.
- Relapse prevention is an integral part of the therapy program.
- Relapse prevention thinking is encouraged, and strategies for relapse prevention are woven into the program from its beginning.
- From the midpoint of therapy (i.e., the point where the offender has developed a heightened awareness of the need not to reoffend), the offender should take part in relapse prevention training, and the emphasis on such training should become increasingly greater as he progresses toward discharge.
- The offender develops a clear understanding of his offending cycle or pattern.

- The offender develops a clear understanding of the relapse process, his most likely routes to relapse, and other possible main routes to relapse.
- The offender recognizes and values the reasons he should stop offending.
- The offender has an active role in developing his relapse prevention plan.
- The offender learns to distinguish between lapse and relapse.
- The offender learns effective coping mechanisms for dealing with lapse.
- The offender learns effective coping mechanisms for dealing with high-risk scenarios, both expected and unexpected.
- The offender recognizes the place of a positive lifestyle in effective relapse prevention.
- The offender plans a realistic and positive offense-free lifestyle.
- The offender makes contingency plans to deal with setbacks and disappointments.
- The offender shares his relapse prevention plan with a network of appropriate people who may act as external monitors.
- The offender attends formal "booster" sessions with those responsible for his therapy at regular intervals after leaving the program.
- The offender has access to professional help after leaving his therapy program.
- Professionals working with the offender apply an antidiscriminatory approach, taking account of the perpetrator's culture and individual considerations such as age, learning abilities, and physical abilities.
- Professionals working with the offender challenge discriminatory attitudes, particularly those associated with sexuality and those linked to sexual offending.
- Those involved in the offender's support/monitoring network work closely together and share information about him openly with each other.

Cycles, Chains, Flowcharts, or Pictures? Providing Links Between the Concepts and Terminology Used in Different Programs

The main aim of relapse prevention for a sex offender is to ensure that he knows his own pattern or patterns, recognizes when he is starting to repeat a pattern, and has plans to deal effectively with that situation. The concepts used to introduce the notion of patterns vary among programs, and the way an offender then works with the concepts is an individual matter. So long as the notion of repetition is communicated, it doesn't matter whether an offender draws a circle, interlinked circles, chains, flowcharts, or other kinds of diagrams and pictures, as long as these make sense to him. One man with whom I worked started explaining his pattern as a jigsaw puzzle, and during his program he hunted for, and found, most of the missing pieces.

In order to engage the offender, it is crucial that the therapist presents him with concepts to which he can relate. The concepts must include recognition that there are individual differences among types of offender and patterns of offending. Key themes include different motivations and beliefs about offending. *Maintaining Change* uses the concept of continuous and inhibited cycles within which thoughts, feelings, and behaviors precede, continue throughout, and follow offending (Eldridge, 1992). Some perpetrators may have continuous cycles based in strong beliefs that sex with adults is good for children. Hence such offenders will not engage with notions of needing to overcome internal inhibitors and being more likely to offend when they're feeling bad.

Some programs use the concept of chains to describe patterns of offending. Ward, Louden, Hudson, and Marshall (1995) describe offense chains, from the first stage of which two subcategories are derived that reflect differing affective states: negative and positive. These influence the subsequent stages. A program that deals only with positive affect pathways would mean very little to a negative-path man, and vice versa. When running groups, it's important to offer the options of different starting points and different sets of beliefs: the lightbulbs visibily go on in offenders' heads when they recognize a pattern like their own.

Maintaining Change is intended to be adaptable for use within a variety of settings; it can provide a link between group and individual work and between prison- and community-based programs of intervention. Although the terminology used differs among programs, the concepts are usually similar or related—hence the exercises in the manual should make sense to most users. The prison program for sexual offenders in England and Wales focuses on the ways in which scenarios, thoughts, and behavior sequences link together to form decision chains. The notion of decision chains is attractive in that it suggests that decision making governs behavior and emphasizes the offender's active role in choosing to take steps leading toward or away from offending.

Probation programs view offenders as having repetitive cycles. These concepts interrelate in that cycles contain numerous decision chains. Some offenders have long-established cycles and understand their patterns best as such. Other offenders have less clear cyclical patterns and may relate better to the idea of decision chains concerning particular sets of events. It is possible to have a decision chain without a cycle. However, the possibility of a repetitive cycle should always be considered. Admission of the existence of a cycle is often difficult for the offender, in that it is suggestive of the possibility of additional offending, hitherto undetected. In deciding which concepts to use, it is important to start where the offender is ready to begin, using the terminology with which he is most familiar.

The traditional relapse prevention literature often refers to *risky situations*, in which the decision to offend is more likely. The term *risky scenario* is used in preference to *risky situation* throughout the personal relapse prevention manual, because *situation* is commonly used to indicate physical circumstances and can be seen by an offender as something external and beyond his control. *Scenario* is a more active term, suggestive of the interplay among thoughts, feelings, and behaviors of different people with each other and with events. However, if an offender prefers to use alternative terminology, so be it. Ultimately, what is important is that the concepts used relate to what actually happens in real life, and that they make sense to the offender.

A Three-Phase Structure Linked to the Intervention Process

Phase 1: From the Beginning to the Midpoint of Therapy

The midpoint of therapy is defined by the offender's progress rather than by actual time. During Phase 1, the offender is introduced to the concept of relapse prevention as part of a statement of the aims of therapy—that is, control rather than cure. The offender is also introduced to monitoring and self-monitoring of change, with an emphasis on self-control and the need for him to understand and break into his own offending pattern. However, during this phase, relapse prevention is an overall, long-term aim. The specific objectives that are the focus of therapy in Phase 1 are concerned with stimulating the offender to recognize the need to change.

Phase 2: From the Midpoint of Therapy Onward

The midpoint is defined here as the point in therapy by which the perpetrator has accepted responsibility for his behavior and is beginning to accept, at an emotional as well as an intellectual level, that the behavior is harmful to himself and/or to others, and that reoffending should be prevented. The offender's development of empathy for his victims is in many cases a key factor in determining his readiness to begin detailed work on relapse prevention.

In this phase, the offender is introduced to relapse prevention strategies. He is helped to identify his routes to relapse and to understand the difference between lapse (i.e., one of the steps toward offending) and relapse (i.e., reoffending itself). He learns to recognize his need to develop mechanisms for dealing with high-risk scenarios, high-risk moods, and lapses. Relapse prevention becomes the central focus of therapy. From this point onward, the offender begins work on the development of an offense-free lifestyle. He uses relapse prevention exercises and techniques to develop a highly individualized plan that will work for him.

Phase 3: After Formal Therapy

The offender is supported when intensive therapy has ended and he has to live the relapse prevention plan. The individualized relapse prevention plan, together with the professionals' specialist knowledge about the relapse process and routes to relapse, are used to focus discussion at call-back sessions or in telephone discussion, as well as for external monitoring by the offender's supporrt network.

The material for use at each phase of the therapy/maintenance process is organized in key areas related to effective relapse prevention. In order for relapse to take place, or be prevented, thoughts, feeings, and actions are required on the part of the perpetrator. Hence, the manual contains exercises which emphasize the need for him to be concerned with each of these aspects of himself.

Note

1. In this guide, the words *perpetrator* and *offender* are used interchangeably to refer to sexual abusers of children. Neither term is intended to imply that the person in question has necessarily been convicted of any crime. Some offenders in relapse prevention programs have been tried for their offenses; many others have not.

Part II

The Change Process

Increasing the Emphasis on Maintenance as the Offender Progresses Through Therapy

Figure 1 displays the change process through which an offender appears to pass in making progress toward an offense-free life. The process is not linear. At times, progress seems rapid, but newborn thinking is fragile and painful, and the offender may slip back into comfortable old ideas before taking the next step forward. The experience of two steps forward and one step back is very common. The change process usually develops as described below.

Word and Thinking Change

The perpetrator admits some offense behavior, and begins to accept responsibility for it. He also begins to develop a conscious understanding of his particular pattern of offending, to recognize that it didn't "just happen." The emphasis of intervention is on challenging the distorted thinking he has developed to legitimate his behavior to himself and others—that is, the thinking he has used to persuade himself that he is not really a sex offender.

At this stage, the offender may start to become aware of the effects of his behavior and to consider the possibility of change. He may hope that someone will provide an answer to his question, "Why do I do this?" and provide him with a neat cure. The message the therapist gives at this point needs to be clear: Control is possible, cure is not. If the offender

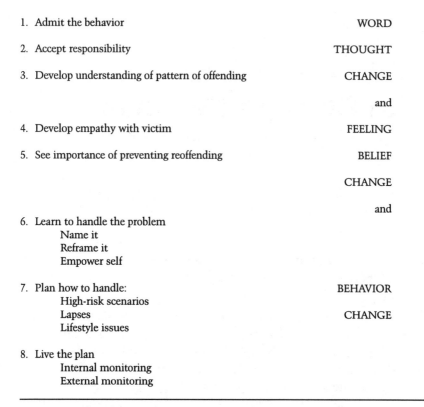

1. Admit the behavior	WORD
2. Accept responsibility	THOUGHT
3. Develop understanding of pattern of offending	CHANGE
	and
4. Develop empathy with victim	FEELING
5. See importance of preventing reoffending	BELIEF
	CHANGE
	and

6. Learn to handle the problem
    Name it
    Reframe it
    Empower self	

7. Plan how to handle:
    High-risk scenarios
    Lapses
    Lifestyle issues
	BEHAVIOR
	
	CHANGE

8. Live the plan
    Internal monitoring
    External monitoring	

Figure 1.   The Change Process

has a cycle that is inhibited for periods of time, he needs to identify the factors that he creates in his life in order to provide himself with an excuse to offend. His fantasy life, both sexual and otherwise, needs to be examined, and, where appropriate, he needs to learn techniques to restructure his fantasies away from offending. He needs to identify his own targeting and grooming behavior so that he will be aware of any such behavior in the future, not only as it applies to children, but also to the significant adults who might take action to prevent children being victimized. The offending behavior itself needs to be reframed as abusive. The place of guilt, if it exists in the offender's cycle, needs to be examined, along with the way the offender deals with guilt feelings in order to escape them and make himself feel better.

The notion that the cycle is being identified so that the offender can learn to break it in the future needs to be introduced early, and the offender encouraged to suggest plans for breaking it. However, until he is beginning to feel and believe, as well as think, that he ought to change, it is unlikely that the offender will have his heart in planning relapse prevention. At this stage, detailed relapse prevention strategies should not be the primary focus of therapy, as the work may too easily provide the offender with a comfortable intellectual exercise in which to escape from the pain of facing the abusive nature of his behavior. As his beliefs about his offending change, the focus on maintenance or relapse prevention will increase.

Feeling and Belief Change

The offender next begins to feel and believe that it is in his own interest to change. He begins to want an offense-free life for himself. He begins to develop empathy for victims, and to feel as well as understand the full impact of his offending at an emotional as well as an intellectual level. If he is a survivor of sexual abuse himself and has previously denied that it harmed him, he may begin to get in touch with his own pain as a victim as well as the pain of his victims. He may begin to see the importance of preventing his reoffending. At this stage he may say, "I'll never do it again," or "I never want to do to another child what was done to me." However, good intentions may not be enough; he needs to plan what course of action he will take when he wants to do it again. He needs to develop strategies to prevent himself from reoffending, so that long-term behavioral change can be sustained.

At this stage, the offender needs to learn how to handle the problem. In the language of Carey and McGrath (1989), he needs to name the urge, reframe it, and empower himself to deal with it. Carey and McGrath suggest that the offender needs to name the urge in order to invoke specific coping mechanisms to identify and deal with high-risk scenarios; he needs to reframe the problem as a learned habitual response, rather than an innate overpowering force; and he needs to empower himself to deal more assertively and less negatively with his life.

If sexual aggression is viewed as the sexual abuse of power, then sex offending can be seen as a maladaptive attempt to cope with feelings of powerlessness and helplessness. The offender experiences the urge to abuse and the consequent pro-offending or offending behavior as an increase in his sense of power. The feeling of being powerful, plus arousal and orgasm to reinforce the feeling, helps explain the intensity of the urge. Hence, in order to reduce his sense of powerlessness and consequently his need to take back power in this way, the offender needs to increase his feeling of being in control of his life generally.

When word and thought change has been joined by some feeling and belief change, the need for maintenance in the form of planning and self-monitoring begins to make sense to the offender, and begins to be developed in therapy.

Most offenders initially want to design plans that emphasize all the things they shouldn't do in order to prevent themselves from doing what they want to do—namely, offending. However, a lifestyle built around "I shouldn't" is unlikely to be effective for long in sustaining change. A plan based on the development of a positive self-image and the replacement of harmful wants by pleasurable nonabusive wants is much more likely to be successful. The offender who says, "I think of the negative consequences every time I want to reoffend, so I know I shouldn't do it" is much more likely to relapse to gratify immediate wants than is the perpetrator who says, "Yes, there are times when I'm still attracted to children, but reoffending doesn't fit with the life I want for myself now." From the beginning, the offender should be encouraged to treat relapse prevention as a positive exercise in which he is discovering the potential gains of giving up offending, rather than focusing on what he feels he has lost.

Behavior Change

Behavior is the great test. Word, thought, feeling, and belief changes are a waste of time without it. However, sustained, as opposed to transitory, behavior change may not happen until the other changes are in place.

When he has the will to pursue an offense-free life, the offender is at a point where he needs to plan how to handle high-risk scenarios, lapses, and lifestyle issues and to begin to change not only long-held beliefs and thinking patterns, but behavior as well. At this stage, the emphasis of intervention needs to be on planning for maintenance of an offense-free life.

If the offender is to live his plan over the long term, he must own it, and it must be tailor-made to his particular offending pattern and lifestyle issues. He becomes an active participant in the creation of his relapse prevention plan, with the therapist acting as facilitator and monitor. Even when sex offenders have worked well in therapy, they are notoriously poor at seeking help from external sources at times of lapse, unless prompted to do so by those acting as external monitors (Pithers, Martin, & Cumming, 1989). Therefore, the plan needs to be shared with appropriate people in a designated network, so that external as well as internal monitoring can take place.

Monitoring the Offender's Progress

Offenders in therapy often learn to say the "right" things before they actually believe them and carry them out; this is to be expected. If an offender is making real progress, however, his beliefs and actions will become congruent with what he says. Wherever possible, his actual behavior needs to be monitored on a regular basis. As Salter (1992) asks, "Is he just talking the talk, or is he walking the walk?"

Regular reviews by those working with the offender in therapy and those who interact with him outside therapy are invaluable. In a residential or prison setting, the review process should include those who have the opportunity to observe the offender outside of therapy when he's off his guard. In a nonresidential therapy setting, the reviews of people who actually live with the offender and/or who are part of his outside monitoring network should be included whenever possible.

In reviews, achievable goals should be set for the offender, and systems set in place for monitoring his progress. So long as the goals are appropriate, they might be quite simple. Other, more complex goals might include the offender's behavior in relation to family members. Whether goals are simple or complex, workable systems need to be in place to monitor the offender's behavior.

In addition to observations of behavior, changes in attributional style should be observed in a systematic way. For example, an offender who is still saying something like "A boy came up to me in the street and asked me the time—I felt really threatened" is clearly still seeing himself in a passive role. An offender who says, "A boy came up to me in the street and asked me the time—I realized I could be a threat to him, so I walked away" has recognized himself as potentially active in the scenario.

Monitoring and evaluation of the offender's progress needs to be an integral part of therapy, with the offender himself and those associated with him having involvement in the process.

Self-Monitoring Using Videotapes

If relapse prevention is to be effective, the offender needs to acquire the habit of checking on his own thoughts, feelings, and behaviors, remembering how these relate to his cycle or pattern of offending. This work should start early and should continue throughout therapy and even after formal therapy ends. Some self-monitoring devices the offender can use include diaries and regularly repeated exercises.

Videotaped monitoring processes can be useful for self-monitoring and for discussion in individual and group therapy. The following two kinds of exercises have worked well as an integral part of therapy (Eldridge & Wyre, 1997):

- *"Breaking the cycle" videotapes:* structured exercises specifically focused on the cycle and how to break it
- *Other self-awareness videotapes:* unstructured exercises in which the perpetrator describes, however he wishes, what he has learned about himself

Both kinds of exercises can be completed at regular intervals, but not necessarily at the same time, to fit in with the therapy program and its particular progress review system. The format we have used is described below.

"Breaking the Cycle" Videos

First session. The first time the perpetrator makes a "breaking the cycle" video, he begins by identifying his cycle in detail: showing his behavioral, thinking, and senses/feeling cycles. He then outlines plans for breaking his cycle. This exercise introduces the offender to the notion of relapse prevention and provides information about his current thinking. After the offender completes the video, he shares it with his therapist and/or group for both positive feedback and constructive criticism. When he makes his first video, the offender is likely to make unrealistic plans that rely primarily on other people behaving according to his wishes.

The perpetrator is unlikely to be aware of his routes to relapse at this stage. Hence, if possible, the first video should include a "last-ditch" plan. This should be something simple, but powerful—a physical action to break away from an immediate desire to offend.

Repeat "breaking the cycle" videos. As the offender moves through therapy, he continues to make "breaking the cycle" videos at regular intervals, until he has a fully developed, workable plan. As he learns more about himself, he may wish to add information about his cycle. However, the main purpose of the subsequent videos is for the offender to make new plans for maintaining the positive changes being made in therapy, and then to describe them coherently so that he can explain them to his support network members—that is, the particular noncollusive people who will support the perpetrator over the long term in his plan for an offense-free life.

Videotape is useful for such exercises because it is equally effective for literate perpetrators and those with literacy problems. A tape can be replayed as necessary, and the offender can hear and see himself verbalizing his intentions whenever he needs to.

As the offender progresses in therapy, his plan for breaking his cycle should include proposed changes in lifestyle and plans for changing his attitudes and beliefs, as well as plans for breaking out of the cycle at all the stages leading up to offending, including last-ditch plans for those times when he is very close to offending despite his good intentions. It should show a clear knowledge of his own cycle, vulnerabilities, and likely routes to relapse, together with knowledge of personal strengths and how he can use these to anticipate, avoid if possible, but primarily deal with lapses. "Breaking the cycle" videotapes are useful both during therapy and on callback after discharge, to ensure that the offender is maintaining an offense-free lifestyle.

The offender should be encouraged to take responsibility for remembering to prepare for and make these videos, so that the idea of self-monitoring becomes a regular part of his lifestyle.

Other Self-Awareness Videotapes

Videotaping can also be useful for other, less structured, self-awareness exercises. The way an offender approaches these exercises provides information about his general level of self-awareness.

The steps toward reoffending may begin so far away from offending itself that the offender doesn't recognize them as having anything to do with his cycle. No one can or should spend his whole life thinking about his cycle of offending. However, a high level of self-awareness can help the offender take action toward maintaining a positive attitude and lifestyle, and thereby reduce his risk of reoffending.

The self-awareness exercise should be as unstructured as possible. The perpetrator should simply be given its title and asked to do whatever he chooses with it.

Psychological Testing

Psychological tests can be employed both before and after formal intervention to assess changes made during the intervention program. These tests are normally concerned with offense-specific issues, such as sexual attitudes and interests, levels of denial and minimization, empathy with victims of abuse, thinking errors related to offending and to children and sexuality, and relapse prevention skills, as well as personality-related issues, such as emotional loneliness, fear of negative evaluation, locus of control, self-esteem, general empathy, and assertiveness. In a study conducted in Great Britain, Beckett, Beech, Fisher, and Fordham (1994) used a battery of normed tests covering these areas to test offenders pre- and post-treatment. A successful treatment effect was related to the extent to which the men reached the normal, nonoffending profile. The measures used by these researchers are listed in Appendix A of this volume. The Relapse Prevention Questionnaire and Interview, presented in Appendix B, was developed by Beckett, Fisher, Mann, and Thornton (1996) from a relapse prevention questionnaire used in this study.

The programs studied by Beckett et al. (1994) were based on a cognitive behavioral approach to treatment. These authors comment:

> This approach targets a number of areas as important in the treatment of sex offenders including promoting victim empathy, reducing distorted thinking, reducing denial and minimisation, developing an awareness of the pattern of offending, developing strategies to deal with deviant arousal, developing alternatives to offending and developing the skills to cope appropriately with situations in which an offence is more likely to occur. Thus in order to evaluate the programmes' effectiveness, measures were used that would detect change in each of the target areas. The measures

chosen focused on the following areas: the offender's level of social
inadequacy, attitude to offending and towards their victim(s), overall
willingness to admit to the extent of their offending, level of distorted
thinking, personality type and relapse prevention techniques. A detailed
personal history was also carried out with each subject, to collect demo-
graphic details including offence history and own victimisation experiences. (p. 53)

Beckett et al. (1994) recognized that sex offenders often lie about their
offending and try to present themselves in ways they believe will be seen
as socially desirable. Hence they included measures to deal with this
problem. They note that "a number of lie scales and social desirability
measures were inserted throughout all the measures and then correlated
with each other" (p. 53). Hanson, Cox, and Woszcyna (1991) also
discuss the importance of such measures in their review of questionnaires for sexual offenders.

Change needs to be monitored at regular intervals during therapy.
One useful test that might be employed in residential or secure programs
is the Behavior Ratings Checklist, devised by the British Prison Core Sex
Offender Treatment Programme. This instrument assesses behavior
outside of formal therapy to see how far treatment change is reflected
in behaviors in other settings. Additionally, Hogue (1992) has developed
the Individual Clinical Rating Form for the prison program. This
instrument, completed monthly, is designed to measure change in
offense-related areas.

Psychophysiological Assessment

Offenders' self-reports concerning their sexual arousal levels to abusive behaviors can be highly inaccurate. Perkins (1995) comments, "As
well as helping the offender accept his sexual interest patterns prior to
treatment, PPG [penile plethysmograph] assessments can also be useful
in monitoring treatment and, in combination with other data, provide
some pointers to possible future risk factors" (p. T37). Perkins cites
Abel, Mittelman, and Becker (1985), who found that self-reported sexual
interest and PPG results coincided in only 30% of offenders assessed,
even when complete confidentiality was assured. When the remaining
70% of the offenders were confronted with this discrepancy, 70% of these
(i.e., 49% of the total sample) revised their self-reports in the direction

of the PPG assessment. The Abel Assessment (Abel, 1995), in which the offender completes a questionnaire and views slides of clothed adults, teenagers, and children, uses the time interval between stimulus onset and offset (i.e., how long the offender views the stimulus) to assess sexual interest; it is less intrusive than the PPG and has similar uses.

Part III

The Phases of Change Linked to the Exercises in *Maintaining Change: A Personal Relapse Prevention Manual*

This part of the therapist's guide is structured to reflect the three phases described in *Maintaining Change: A Personal Relapse Prevention Manual,* and should be read in conjunction with that manual. The discussion provides rationales for the exercises in the manual as well as practice-based ideas for working with the material.

Phase 1

From the Beginning to the Midpoint of Therapy

Phase 1 for therapists links with the Phase 1 material in the personal relapse prevention manual (Manual, pp. 1-33), which is intended to motivate the perpetrator to identify his own pattern in detail. Working with some of the blocks to program receptivity, and ways of introducing and using the exercises are described in this section. The exercises can be given to the perpetrator all at once or individually, at the therapist's discretion.

NOTE: Manual page numbers refer to pages in *Maintaining Change: A Personal Relapse Prevention Manual.*

During Phase 1, it is important that the offender recognize that the aim of therapy is self-control rather than cure. For offenders who are living in the community, some work on relapse prevention may need to take place immediately. Where possible, detailed work on relapse prevention techniques is better placed in Phase 2, after the perpetrator has developed some level of empathy for his victims (see Part II of this volume).

The building of a network of key people to support and monitor the offender needs to start during Phase 1, and ways of doing this are discussed in the manual. In cases where the offender has abused a member or members of his own family, parallel work may need to begin at an early stage.

Motivating Offenders: Working With Blocks to Receptivity

The Phase 1 handout "Learning Control" and the exercises "Is Offending Really So Great?" and "Gains and Losses of Reoffending for You" (Manual, pp. 2-5) are intended to motivate offenders to analyze critically the place of offending in their lives. They can be used to open discussions about the blocks to change and to reveal what factors may prevent an offender from being receptive to the intervention program. Blocks to offender receptivity can include fear of the consequences of complete disclosure, fear of change, unresolved childhood victim experiences, fear of feelings, negative thinking, and a highly disordered arousal pattern. Ways of overcoming each of these are considered below.

Fear of the Consequences of Complete Disclosure

Most sex offenders do not give complete information during initial assessment because they fear that if the scale of their offending and their responsibility for it are divulged, they will go to prison, lose their families, be beaten up by the neighbors—in short, they will be rejected by everyone, perhaps including themselves. The therapist needs to recognize the offender's fear of the consequences of disclosure and create a positive environment where he feels that it's okay to talk. Offenders are often anxious about whether their therapists will be shocked. Stating your experience in the work can be very enabling. Previously anxious offenders have said to me, "So you've heard it all before," with a note of relief in their voice, and then disclosed more information.

Fear of consequences of disclosure is often unjustified. A man's wife may realize that he is guilty, and the child protection agencies may believe he is guilty and be prepared to work with him, if he tells the truth—but not if he doesn't. Recognizing his dilemma and then helping him work out the pros and cons of giving information can be a way for the therapist to unstick a stuck situation. Process commenting helps move interviews forward; for example, the therapist might say, "I guess you must be worried about what to tell me and what might happen if you do."

Working with "if" can also be very helpful. For example, I said to one man: "Only you and the child know what actually happened. I don't, but I have worked with lots of people who did do it and are denying everything that happened because they're understandably worried about the consequences. If you were in that position, what might get in the way of you telling?" Hypothetical questions can go further: "If you had done it, what might your reason have been?" "How would you have done it?" "How might you have persuaded her to go along with it?"

Gaining rapport is vital to engaging the perpetrator (Eldridge & Wyre, in press). Talking with a perpetrator about the need to develop rapport can aid that process. Make explicit that you're going to test out assumptions based on knowledge of sex offending, and say, "Please tell me if I get it wrong."

Motivating offenders is about encouragement. Attach positives to perceived negatives. For example, my colleague Ray Wyre once asked an offender a question about fantasy. The man replied, "I don't fantasize!" Instead of disputing this, Ray said, "I mean thoughts. Clearly you thought about it before you did it, and that's good because it shows how much control you have." It is useful for the therapist to give positive feedback to the offender for his first tentative steps forward. Talking about what he has done and his own responsibility for it may be the most difficult thing he has ever had to do. A negative reception will close him down, perhaps forever.

It is productive for the therapist to engage in a partnership with the offender, the aim of which is to explore together what the offender did and what he can do to change. Some of the interviewing approaches discussed by Jenkins (1990) and Miller and Rollnick (1991) can aid in this process. Jenkins offers ways of inviting men to "attend to the abuse" (p. 120) in cases of different levels of denial of responsibility, including total denial. He emphasizes the need for the therapist at the beginning of contact to recognize openly some of the man's feelings and fears and then to attach positives to the man facing up to his responsibility: "Facing up offers the only way that a man can develop some self-respect and learn to live with himself instead of living a lie and being constantly on the run from himself" (p. 129). A key theme throughout Jenkins's approach is the affirmation and harnessing of the offender's positive qualities for change.

A therapeutic group environment is also vital. In both the residential programs I have run with colleagues, we formally introduced each new offender member of the group to our principles for providing a noncollusive but safe place for change. The essence of this is that we share information in the interests of protecting children; we care for the offenders, but that's different from trusting them; we challenge with respect; we emphasize what is good about them; we aim to give hope for change, and that can come only from honest rather than conning relationships; and we believe in control rather than cure (Eldridge & Wyre, 1997). Taking the temperature of intervention groups on a regular basis is a valuable way of checking that the culture continues to be conducive to change. The Group Environment Scale (Moos, 1986) is a useful tool for this purpose.

Fear of Change

Many perpetrators have built their lives around offending and fear that if they change they'll lose everything that matters to them. This is especially true of preferential pedophiles, who have strong emotional congruence with children and fear the loneliness that might result if they lose children in their lives. They also fear loss of the only sexual and fantasy life they've ever known. In order for change to become attractive, it must include positive non-abusive alternatives. Without this there will be an unsustainable vacuum.

Unresolved Childhood Victim Experiences

Offenders who were extensively victimized as children and who tried to take power back by believing that they, not their abusers, were in control, often develop distorted but logical beliefs based on their experience. One man who was abused by a group of pedophiles when he was young said, "It happened to me as a child; I liked it, it did me no harm.

My victims aren't really victims either; they're willing partners, like I was." If that belief remains, it is impossible for him to get off the starting blocks in therapy. Fear of giving up such beliefs is strong, too. One man said to me, "I'm afraid of what I'll lose if I change." His fears were about losing his perceptions of family relationships. To face the fact that the people who you believed loved you were really exploiting and abusing you requires a very safe environment.

For such men, work focusing on their childhood victim experiences may be required before they can begin to work on their offending. Some therapists express the fear that this can lead to men developing insight into why they offend and abdicating responsibility for their offending. The therapist can avoid this situation by helping the offender make links. For example:

> Sam was abused at age 10 by George. Sam is now 40 and has abused John, who is 10. Sam's therapist focused on how Sam wasn't responsible for what George did to him when he was a child, and then linked that to how Sam must be responsible for his offending against John, because John surely wasn't responsible any more than Sam had been when he was a child. In getting in touch with his own pain and nonresponsibility as a child, Sam got in touch with his victim's pain and nonresponsibility.

Fear of Feelings

Offenders who have unresolved experiences in their own past are often fearful of recognizing and dealing with their own painful feelings. They may be afraid of working on the role of feelings in their cycle for this reason. It is helpful to talk about this at an early stage and to suggest that a plan be devised for managing painful feelings. If therapy is to be effective, it is important that the offender allow himself to stay with those feelings for a time, but has mechanisms for managing them. If he has not, then he may avoid the feelings altogether, or experience them, panic or become depressed and revert to old dysfunctional cycle-related ways of coping. Effective plans include activities which are stress-free and have no association with sex or with offending. The more action based they are, the more likely they are to work. This approach has the dual benefit of increasing receptivity to the program and introducing offenders to the relapse prevention concept of developing effective effective coping mechanisms to deal with mood-state routes to relapse.

Negative Thinking

One very common block to receptivity, especially among offenders who have obviously fragile personalities, but sometimes among seemingly more secure people, is negative thinking. Negative thinking can relate to other areas of vulnerability, such as low self-esteem, under-assertiveness, poor anger management, and inclination toward depression.

If assessment of an offender has identified a fear of negative evaluation or a tendency for him to fall into a pattern of feeling bad about himself, expecting rejection, seeing rejection even when it's not there, behaving in ways that invite rejection, unassertiveness, withdrawal into comforting fantasy (often offense related), and finding excuses to reoffend, then it may be useful to start work on the manual's Phase 2 handout titled "Changing Your Thoughts and Feelings" (Manual, pp. 102-105), and do the related exercises at an early stage in therapy. These can help the offender to identify the self-talk that takes him through his negative pattern and the kind of generalized thinking errors that may be present. A person with this kind of pattern may perceive very minor criticisms or casual remarks made by others as signs of total rejection, not just by the individuals speaking, but by the whole adult human race. This can lead him from unrealistic negative thinking about himself in relation to other adults to distorted "false positive" thinking about children (e.g., "Only children understand me").

When an offender learns to challenge his own negative thoughts, his ability to accept criticism positively is increased. This can also help him move to a position where he dares to feel empathy for his victims. Often, the fear of what it will mean to accept challenge can prevent a man from being receptive. The underlying thought, "If I did that wrong, then there's nothing good about me; I should kill myself," can effectively prevent him from entertaining the possibility that he might have done something wrong.

In encouraging an offender to challenge negative thinking, the therapist must emphasize that realistic positive thinking, not false positive thinking, is the way forward. A good example of false positive thinking is "I shouldn't give myself a hard time; the child liked it, really." Realistic positive thinking might be "Yes, that was a bad thing I did, and I'm capable of good things too."

Many offenders find bibliotherapy helps them think more positively. *Feeling Good* by David Burns (1981) is written for anyone who has ever wanted to think more positively, including therapists! It has been very effective in changing generalized negative thinking patterns with many offenders who have included it in their Relapse Prevention Collections.

A Highly Disordered Arousal Pattern

A high level of arousal to thoughts of offending and a fantasy life strongly focused on offending can render therapy ineffective. It may be necessary to begin to work on controlling sexual arousal levels and patterns prior to going on to further work. In some cases, behavioral techniques such as covert sensitization or masturbatory satiation should be started at an early stage (Beckett, 1994).

Working With Multidimensional Cycles of Sex Offending

The Phase 1 handouts and exercises relating to sex offending cycles aim to help perpetrators identify their own cycles. In order to start this process, they are introduced to the way cycles can operate, together with examples of components of non-offending and offending cycles, with which they work interactively. In recognizing the patterns of Ray and Walter, the fictional characters in the exercises, they begin to identify their own patterns, including some of the seemingly irrelevant decisions which led to offending and the thoughts and moods that preceded it.

Phase 1 material can be given to the perpetrators prior to groupwork on sex offending cycles, but is more useful after group discussion. Start groups with a brief discussion of the cycle process, and then encourage group members to brainstorm the thoughts that constitute pro-offending thinking, the way that fantasy works, who they target, and how they groom people. The more participatory and the less didactic the experience, the more able group members will be to work out their own patterns of offending. Techniques for helping perpetrators identify their thinking, feeling, and senses cycles are described in this section.

Common Patterns

Men who sexually abuse children are not a homogeneous group. They have different motivations, different personality types, different levels of fixation, and different modi operandi. They come from all walks of life. Salter (1995, p. 29) notes that Maletzky (1991) "concluded in his sample of more than 5000 sex offenders that"

> there has been no documentation of a typical "offender personality." . . . Rather, these men were characterized by their diversity: An offender could as well have been a professor as a pauper, a minister as an atheist, a teetotaler as an alcoholic, a teenager as a septuagenarian. Moreover, an offender . . . might as well have had an extensive history of arrests or none at all, and might as well have had associated diagnoses as none. . . . In retrospect, these patients did not seem to share any definable demographic or personality traits to render them distinctive. (pp. 16-17)

However, one feature commonly found among perpetrators of child sexual abuse whose behavior has come to the notice of the courts is that, in most cases, they have been offending against either an individual victim or multiple victims for some time. In many instances a repetitive cycle has developed, although there may be times when it is not active. Identification of the cycle and the way it operates within the offender's life, as he moves through nonoffending periods into relapse, is a major task of intervention and relapse prevention.

Throughout the offender's cycle, distorted thinking is apparent. The offender holds beliefs that give him permission to offend; he legitimates, excuses, minimizes, or justifies his behavior, or blames someone else for it. There are usually phases during which he fantasizes about offending, plans to offend, and targets and grooms both the victim and other people to prevent disclosure. These phases occur in most sex offending cycles, but the modi operandi within the phases vary depending on the type of perpetrator. For example, an anger-motivated rapist who abuses children and adults may have different thinking patterns and may use tactics very different from those used by a professional pedophile. Both have beliefs that facilitate their behavior, and both target and groom their victims, but their beliefs and their tactics are quite different. The way in which the cycle starts depends on the beliefs and arousal patterns of the offender. As Salter (1995) notes:

The deviant cycle is generally triggered by (a) an affective state, such as rage, anxiety, depression, or boredom; (b) a chronically disordered sexual arousal pattern in which the offender is sexually attracted to children or to violence; or (c) an antisocial attitude in which the offender is willing to use anyone or anything for sexual gratification and for fulfillment of his need to have power and control over others. (pp. 51-52)

During his cycle, the offender is often good at self-delusion: He convinces himself that there is no planning and that things just happen. The speed at which the cycle progresses varies enormously among perpetrators. Some go through lengthy periods of preparation; others go very quickly from the thought to the offense.

Cycles are not unique to sex abuse perpetrators. Most people who are trying to cut down on or give up something they enjoy know all about selective thinking, seemingly irrelevant decision making, and how on a bad day, self-delusion increases and the likelihood of relapse is greater. However, although the process may be very common, in the case of a sex abuse perpetrator the content, or desired behavior, is often extremely bizarre. Hence, in order to legitimate it, he has to indulge in highly distorted thinking.

Motivation and Core Beliefs

Motivations vary among individual perpetrators, but they serve a common purpose: to justify, excuse, or legitimate the behavior. Some examples of perpetrators' comments about their offending are illustrative:

- Joe, who abused young children, said, "When I see a child who seems happy, I'm jealous and I want to take their childhood away and hurt them like I was hurt. I never had a childhood."
- Bob, on the other hand, told himself, "It happened to me when I was a child and I enjoyed it. It did me no harm, it'll do them no harm. It's not abuse." Bob worked hard at persuading both himself and the children that "this is love. It's not abuse, it's normal, it's just the law that's wrong."
- Mike, a stepfather who abused both out of anger and when he wanted comfort and affection, said, "I just make them think what I think, and that's 'I want and I take.' "
- John, who abused most of the children in his family network, was much more interested in completing a sexual act involving oral

abuse than he was in a particular type of person. Anyone would do; his victims were simply his blowup dolls.

- Sam, a man who primarily abused girls around puberty and believed that postpubescent girls are provocative, saw his behavior as socially, if not legally, acceptable and saw no reason to question it. He abused his stepdaughter, explaining the abuse by saying, "It was the way she dressed that made me do it; and she's got a real sexy body—what could a man do?"

Belief Systems Producing Continuous or Inhibited Cycles

Whatever the type of offender, cycles seem to be either continuous or inhibited, depending on the basic attitudes and beliefs the offender holds and the strength of his desire to offend. It is important when assessing an offender, to identify his individual pattern or patterns, rather than force-fitting him into a general category. However, as a starting point, it is useful to understand some of the differences between continuous and inhibited cycles (see Figure 2).

Continuous Cycles

Offenders with continuous cycles have belief systems that legitimate their behavior to the point where the cycle is only interrupted by their perceived risk of being caught. For example, a fixated pedophile who believes sexual abuse is not abuse at all, but an expression of love, may convince himself that he's really helping or "loving" children. A man who believes that postpubertal girls are generally provocative and "ask for it" may persuade himself that they deserve or want "it."

Breaks in the cycles of such offenders will occur only if they discover that they have made a targeting error; for example, the child they have chosen may tell, and is therefore too risky to pursue. In this case, they may target another child or children. Such offenders have an essentially continuous cycle, uninterrupted by worries about the way their behavior harms either their own self-image or their victims.

These offenders have extremely distorted beliefs about their offending behavior, and they will delude themselves about their victims' behavior, interpreting it in ways that support their beliefs. However, they do not delude themselves about the process by which they come to offend. When detected, they may lie to the police and the courts, pretending that their offending "just happened once," but they do not lie to

CONTINUOUS CYCLE

INHIBITED CYCLE

"SHORT-CIRCUIT" CYCLE

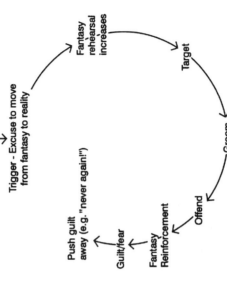

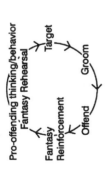

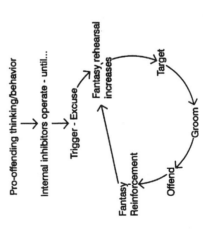

Figure 2. Continuous, Inhibited, and "Short-Circuit" Cycles

themselves about the premeditated and deliberate nature of their offending, because they believe that right is really on their side.

Inhibited Cycles

Offenders who have inhibited cycles do question their own behavior. They see it as essentially perverted and worry about the way it reflects on them. They may also recognize that it hurts their victims. These offenders have internal inhibitors that operate to break their cycles. The length of the breaks depends on the strength of (a) the internal inhibitors, (b) the distorted or pro-offending thinking that legitimates offending, and (c) the arousal or desire to offend.

Some offenders have quite lengthy periods when their cycles are inhibited and they do not offend. However, they still indulge in thoughts that legitimate offending, and they may still fantasize about abuse, thereby strengthening their desire to reoffend. They may also reinforce their own distorted thinking about abuse by, for example, fantasizing about rape in which the victim resists at first but ends up enjoying it, or in which children smile and say, "Please do it to me."

Such offenders may seek excuses to offend. They may make a whole series of seemingly irrelevant decisions leading to the opportunity to carry out the secretly desired behavior. This process enables them to avoid facing the pain and responsibility of recognizing that they planned to reoffend.

Other offenders may break through their internal inhibitors by indulging in self-fulfilling prophecies that lead them to feel sorry for themselves and entitled to comfort. For example, an offender with a poor self-image, whether owing to past experiences or to his identification of himself as a pervert, may expect other people to realize he is "no good" and reject him. He sees rejection even if it's not there, by seeing and hearing selectively. He may then behave in ways that create rejection. Hence he eventually sees that the world is against him, and this provides him with an excuse to seek comfort in his own distorted beliefs. He may fantasize increasingly about children, using as justification the belief that only children love and understand him, while the adult world does not.

Another offender who perceives rejection may indulge in revenge-type fantasies about attacking and hurting others because he feels attacked and hurt. Sometimes fantasies may include distorted "love" and revenge components. Offenders who tell themselves they love children may, for example, also be motivated by anger. Essentially, though, the offender is interpreting external events and the behavior of others in a distorted way, thus providing himself with a distorted rationale to do what he wants—namely, to reoffend.

Having begun offending again after a period of abstinence, some perpetrators feel guilty and may not reoffend further for periods of time ranging from a few days to several years. However, as their core beliefs have not changed, and at some level they still wish to reoffend, they may relapse by repeating the pattern.

Short-Circuiting the Phases of an Inhibited Cycle

Some offenders are inclined to "short-circuit" once they start reoffending. Some go into "binge mode." They feel they have failed and so give up trying to avoid offending, or drown their sorrows in further fantasy and offending, which temporarily makes them feel better. In some cases, alcohol abuse may become part of the cycle, to provide "Dutch courage" before offending and to drown guilt and self-pity afterward. Essentially, these perpetrators reoffend to push away the pain of having reoffended.

Short-circuiting of the various phases of the cycle may also appear when an offender has targeted and groomed one particular victim or group of victims. For example, an offender who abuses within a family will have groomed the victim to comply without telling, and will have groomed family relationships in such a way that the abuse is unlikely to be discovered. Hence he no longer needs to target the victim, and the odd tweak on the strings of those he is seeking to control is all that is required to keep his offending secret. He may push away guilt feelings by telling himself that his daughter would have told someone if she really minded. He conveniently forgets that he has told her that discovery would kill her mother.

Eventually, content in the belief that he has a consenting, if secret, relationship, he no longer needs to fantasize much either. He arranges when he will be able to abuse, and he simply goes from the thought to the offense.

Linked Cycles

Some offenders have continuous cycles in relation to one set of sexual behaviors and/or victims and inhibited cycles in relation to others. For example, an offender may truly believe it is acceptable to behave sexually toward a postpubertal child, but may believe it is abusive to behave sexually toward a younger child. The thinking that enables him to abuse the older child without question may, over time, erode his belief that he should not abuse the younger child. If it is good for the older child, why not for the younger as well? Offenders who abuse their stepchildren regularly and without question may use this same distorted logic to legitimate the abuse of their own children.

Permission-Giving
Thinking Errors in Fantasy

Thoughts and sexual fantasies about abuse usually precede action. In fantasy anything goes: The would-be perpetrator can imagine a rape in which the victim resists at first but ends up enjoying it, or a child who smiles and says, "Please do it to me." Fantasy acts as a disinhibitor and as a reinforcer, and allows the offender to picture the child of his choice doing what he wishes. Barry, an abuser of both girls and boys, talked about "putting the mask of my fantasy on to the real-life child." Walking down the street with Mary, the 6-year-old child of a friend, he would feel her take his hand, as children do. Privately, he had fantasized about her and put a "please have sex with me" meaning onto this simple action. When Mary holds his hand in real life, he transfers the fantasy meaning across; hence she and her reality become invisible to Barry. Later, when he has abused Mary, he may be very convincing when he says to her, "But you shouldn't have held my hand if you hadn't wanted it."

Targeting Behaviors

Having begun to fantasize about abuse, the offender begins to plan, target a child and groom, or manipulate, both the intended victim and anyone who may protect the victim. The essence of choosing safely and grooming effectively is the offender's persuasion of the child that it is "something about you that made me do it." The essence of manipulating those who might protect the victim is to persuade them that "I am not the sort of person who would do these things" or, failing that, "It's your fault if I did these things, and hence you can't tell."

Offenders don't just target any children; they also aim to choose a child from a family in which they can exert control. Shaun, a priest who offended against boys, chose boys from families where there were tensions. Brian, a teacher, chose boys from families to which he could offer much-needed help with employment and personal problems. Michael, a pedophile, chose boys who had weak relationships with their fathers.

Offenders frequently choose children from their own families, as this usually allows the greatest scope for control because of issues relating to trust and dependency. For example, Imran chose his young nephew, who had recently come to live in England with his mother, who spoke no English. Imran had absolute control over both the boy and his mother, who were isolated, confused, and trapped in a new country. Maurice chose the eldest of his three stepdaughters. She had learning difficulties and was already quite isolated from her younger sisters; he developed a special relationship with her, taking an interest in her hobbies and helping her with schoolwork. Warren singled out one of his daughters almost from birth, and fostered a very close relationship with her that allowed no one else near. Sean chose his foster daughter, who had lost her entire family in a house fire.

Offenders are good at convincing their victims that they are being abused because of "something about you." However, the reality is that offenders will use factors far outside the control of either the children or their families in order to create vulnerability. They will home in on normal, ordinary human problems and use these to gain access and control. It's not "something about you," it's more likely to be something about the way the offender looks for and uses circumstances.

Grooming: Manipulative Tactics to Gain Compliance and Prevent Disclosure

Whatever their motivations or belief systems, most offenders have in common the use of highly manipulative tactics to control their victims and other people who might recognize and reveal their offending. Tactics used to control vary among offenders. Both the sadistic offender, who wishes to hurt and cause pain to children, and the fixated pedophile, who pretends he loves children, use tactics to control their victims, but the tactics and their effects are very different.

Offenders manipulate both children and those who could protect them. The tactics they use include overt physical violence, threats of violence, bribes, emotional dependency, and often a combination of all of these. The "Jekyll and Hyde" approach ("I can be loving and kind, but if you don't do what I say, you'll see my teeth!") is very common.

Grooming the Child

For many offenders, the main purpose of grooming the child is to make the child carry the burden of guilt. Offenders make blame shifting into a distorted art form. The following are some offenders' descriptions of the tactics they have used to imply their victims' complicity and to threaten and control the children they abused. The same themes arise repeatedly:

"I give them things: money, presents."

"I give them a false sense of responsibility. I share adult things with them. I took them with me when I did other illegal things, I taught them, you never say anything about these things, never mention them—and that includes the sex side. You can only be treated as grown up when you learn to keep your mouth shut; it's the law of the criminal fraternity, and you have to learn it if you want to stay safe. I'm trusting you to do that. If you say anything about any of this I'll go to prison."

"I teach them keeping secrets is okay."

"You get them to believe you're a friend."

"You make them believe you love them."

"You make them believe they love you."

"I make them feel adult feelings is all right for them to feel; feeling good about sex is okay, you don't have to be an adult to feel good about sex. If you feel good about it, then just go with it."

"Make them dependent."

"Make them think they need you."

"Create a false sense of security."

"Teach them 'Daddy knows best.' "

"If they disobey me they'll get tellings off and good hidings."

"You make them aware that adults around you are frightened of you; show the power you have over other adults, just by the presence you put across. If they think adults are frightened of you and won't argue with you, they'll think, 'What chance have I got?' You don't threaten the child, but you threaten adults while the child's there. It's intimidation, really."

"Say, 'No one will believe you.' "

"Say, 'You'll get into trouble and be taken away from home.' "

"Say, 'If I go, your good life goes.' "

"Say, 'If I go, who's going to buy you these things?' "

"Tell them, 'It'll kill your mother if she finds out.' "

Grooming Nonabusing Parents

The following quotes from offenders show some common tactics they use to control the parents of children they abuse:

"Be nice to them; get yourself to be trusted."

"Say you love and care for the children and get them to see that."

"Make love to her [the children's mother], show love and affection toward her."

"Be helpful."

"Corruption of the mother: Show provocative love and affection in front of the children and say it's just part of growing up for the children to see you with an erection."

"Using what you know to threaten, saying, 'If you tell, I'll tell everyone about . . .' "

"She [the children's mother] knows I can be loving and she knows I can be angry and violent."

One man manipulated both his wife and stepdaughter in a way that effectively prevented disclosure for many years. He set up his stepdaughter to be thought a liar, and then abused her, using aggressive tactics to frighten her into silence. When his wife came home from work shortly afterward, he would "make love to her." He planned that if his stepdaughter did disclose, her mother might think, "How could he possibly have done this (a) at all, (b) just before making love to me? I know my daughter lies and wishes I hadn't married him—she's making this up to get rid of him."

Offenders often divert the victim's anger onto the nonabusing parent and encourage the victim to believe that the other parent knows about the abuse or is in some way to blame. An offender may achieve this by being aggressive toward the nonabusing parent but seemingly loving to the child he is abusing, or by behaving like a child with the children and setting his partner up to be the disciplinarian.

The Guilty Phase

As noted above, the guilty phase experienced by an offender with an inhibited cycle after he commits acts of abuse may break the cycle in the short term, but it can actually feed the cycle in the longer term, as the offender tries to push away uncomfortable feelings. Many offenders describe how they use fantasy in order to feel better. Over time, they learn that this provides immediate, if short-lived, comfort and gratification. As has been seen, a comforting fantasy usually involves highly distorted thinking; for example, the perpetrator visualizes children asking for and enjoying sex with him, or being physically hurt and miraculously surviving unscathed. Essentially, the offender confirms the distorted beliefs that legitimate his abusive behavior, and this enables the pattern to be repeated.

Thinking, Feeling, and Senses Cycles

In the early stages, it is often helpful in challenging denial to have a very behavior-specific focus. If the therapist makes and tests assumptions about behavior and enables the offender to talk about the what, where, who, and how of the offense scenario, this can greatly facilitate disclosure.

When the offender begins to identify his own pattern and to face the reality of his own planning of events and his manipulation of the victim and other people to maintain the secret, then he will appropriately focus on his own behavior at all the stages. If he has an inhibited cycle, he will also begin to recognize the process of self-delusion whereby he allows himself to believe that he isn't really planning to offend; he will begin to analyze the seemingly irrelevant decisions that have led to seemingly irrelevant pieces of behavior, which collectively have led to reoffending.

In this way, he may begin to recognize that the cycle isn't just about behavior—it is also about thoughts. At this stage it can be helpful for him to try to remember the thoughts he had before, during, and after one particular offense. If he can then repeat this exercise in relation to a number of different offenses, he may be able to recognize a pattern. These recollections provide crucial information for use in therapy and in relapse prevention work. They are thoughts and thought patterns that the perpetrator himself needs to learn to challenge and to recognize as risk signs in the future.

The recognition of a thinking cycle can stimulate the identification of feelings cycles. Although negative thoughts often exacerbate negative feelings, the feelings themselves may be triggered by other negative thoughts, or by physiological disturbance initially triggered by environmental stimuli. It is important that the offender learns to recognize the feelings that precipitate a greater desire to offend. In some cases, for example, where these relate to his own unresolved victim experiences, it may be helpful for him to address the origins of such feelings in therapy. Such work may be very important, but is unlikely to be so effective that the offender never experiences those feelings again. Hence it is crucial that he learns effective coping mechanisms to deal with them in the future.

Feelings are often the consequence of thoughts or physiological responses to external stimuli, rather than to the stimuli themselves. The meaning placed on a certain stimulus may be based on past experiences, and may not be immediately accessible at a conscious level; hence it seems as if the external stimulus is the direct cause of the changed mood and thought pattern.

Sometimes the scenario is even more confusing: An individual may experience a number of external stimuli simultaneously that remind him of a particular event—perhaps a combination of sights, sounds, and smells. An offender who has good rapport with his therapist can usually identify the senses cycles that match his thought and behavior cycles. This is also crucial information for both therapy and post-therapy phases. The following examples are illustrative of these issues.

Javeed

Javeed's offending followed a rigid pattern. He always approached boys aged about 10 who looked like he did at that age. His approach was identical every time: He would expose himself to the boy. If the boy ran away, Javeed would see him as the "good boy" he, Javeed, should have been when he was a child being abused by adults. If he stayed, then Javeed would assault him, rationalizing this by thinking that the boy must want sex, or he would have run away.

An analysis of Javeed's thinking cycle revealed a lot of issues related to his confusion about his own victim experiences. An analysis of his feeling and senses cycle revealed related unresolved feelings and memories. This analysis was valuable because (a) it greatly facilitated survivor work with Javeed on his own victim experiences; (b) this helped unblock him from failure to empathize with his own victims (although Javeed had taken responsibility for his offending and was aware that his victims didn't consent, he had been slow to develop empathy, perhaps because of fear of getting in touch with his own pain as a victim); and (c) as he learned more about all the dimensions of his cycle, it became easier for Javeed to recognize the development of moods that preceded his offending phases and to take action before he felt swamped by them.

George

George sexually abused his stepdaughter repeatedly over a period of years. He said that he had enjoyed offending and felt good afterward. However, an analysis of his feelings cycle revealed that he had always felt depressed afterward. This obviously had immediate value in therapy.

An analysis of George's senses cycle revealed that as part of grooming prior to offending, George would buy chocolate milk shakes for his stepdaughter. When he had her alone in the house, he would wash both himself and her, as a lead-up to overt sexual abuse. George's wife usually bought a particular brand of soap, and it was this soap that George used. Over time, the smell of this soap became so closely linked with arousal for George that he insisted the family buy only that brand.

The analysis of George's senses cycle was valuable in the following ways. First, it made George conscious of some of the stimuli that hindered his progress. For example, during the time of his therapy, George was still using this particular brand of soap, which made it much more difficult for him to control his desire to masturbate while thinking about abuse. When he became aware of the connection, he changed his brand of soap. Second, having given up using the soap, George had a useful warning signal for future problems. If he caught himself even picking up this brand of soap in the supermarket, he knew that this would be an early warning sign of a slide toward reoffending.

Third, George was now aware of the particular smells that reminded him of offending, and this awareness could protect him from a stimulus overload route to relapse. For example, if, without this self-knowledge, George had been hit all at once by the smell of the soap, the odor of chocolate in some form, and the sight of a child who looked a bit like his stepdaughter, he may have felt a strong desire to offend, without knowing how that came about. It might feel like a bolt from the blue—an overpowering force. If he blamed the feeling on any of the stimuli, it would probably be the child and his own weakness. He might go straight into the thinking error "Children provoke me and I can't resist." With knowledge of the stimuli, George could learn to attach aversive meanings to the smell of chocolate and the soap. Even without this, his knowledge could enable him to recognize what was happening and he could interpret his reactions in ways that gave him control. He could understand what was happening rather than feel mystified and overwhelmed by it. What George tells himself about the source of his physiological arousal is crucial in how he decides to deal with it. (See the section on Phase 2 material for more about the stimulus overload route to lapse and relapse.)

Techniques for Identifying the Senses Cycle

A Three-Stage Model for Homework

To identify the offender's senses cycle, the therapist can ask him to draw out his behavioral cycle first, showing his pattern of offending—that is, how the stages work for him. If he has more than one cycle relating to different children, or if he has linked cycles, ask him to identify these. When he has completed this task in sufficient detail, ask him to think about each stage and identify what his thoughts are at each point. He should then write down his actual thoughts in the first person, and in present tense. For example, upon seeing a likely victim, the offender may think, "He's a possible" or "I think we could be lovers." This exercise can help to identify some of the automatic distorted thinking that helps keep the cycle going.

When the offender has completed the work of writing down the thoughts in his thinking cycle, ask him to identify his "senses and feeling" cycle. For each point in the cycle, he should identify what he saw, heard, smelled, tasted, touched, and felt. If the offender does this work on his own, the therapist should be careful to ensure that he has support. This exercise can be very distressing for offenders who are themselves survivors of abuse. Often the senses and feelings in their cycles relate to their own victim experiences.

"Live" First-Person, Present-Tense Recall

Another method the therapist might use to help the offender access his thoughts and feelings, as well as the role of his senses in his cycle, is to ask him to recall a particular day when he offended. The therapist should provide some introduction to this exercise, explaining that this is a way of helping the offender focus his memory on the lead-up to his offending. It is useful to videotape the session, so that the offender can watch himself afterward and identify his own triggers.

Ask the offender to relax, close his eyes, and try to get back in touch with a particular day, and to remember early in the day, well before he offended. When the offender confirms that he feels he's there, ask him to say where he is, talking in the first person and in present tense. When satisfied that he is describing something that he remembers clearly, the therapist should ask him what he can see, smell, touch, taste, and hear, and what he is thinking and feeling.

Ask what happens next. For example, the offender describes being in the bedroom and identifies what he can see, hear, smell, touch, and taste, and what he is thinking and feeling at the time. When asked what happens next, he replies, "I go downstairs." The therapist says, "Okay, you're going down the stairs, what can you see? [pauses for reply] Hear? [pauses for reply]" and so on.

The therapist continues this process up to the point where the perpetrator is about to commit the offense. There is no need to go through all the details of the offense; it is more useful to move from just before the offense to just afterward. Offenders often feel highly excited before they offend, and depressed and low afterward. This exercise can heighten the offender's awareness of this change, and he may be able to use that awareness in preventing reoffending.

When the exercise has been completed, ask the offender to watch the videotape of the session and identify what he thinks are key senses, thoughts, and moods for him. What are his primary triggers? What works/fails in terms of interrupting the pattern? Sometimes offenders have ideas for relapse prevention that senses cycle work shows are counterproductive in practice. For example, Bartholomew, a vicar, believed that he might be deterred from reoffending if he thought of the police; however, work on his senses/feelings cycle revealed that he became more excited when he drove past the police station.

Senses cycle work is very effective in enhancing an understanding of the way the cycle works. However, the perpetrator can feel very close to offending 'mode' after doing the work, so it's important to ensure that toward the close of the exercise, he is reminded that he was caught, sent to court, and is now attending a program to prevent reoffending. Timing is important too. The work should not be done on a day when there is insufficient time to wind down from it, or when family sessions are planned. If possible, the tape should be analyzed by the offender and therapist immediately after completing it as this helps clarify its purpose and context.

Building Networks: Phase 1

by Hilary Eldridge and Jenny Still

In the Phase 1 material in *Maintaining Change: A Personal Relapse Prevention Manual,* the offender is introduced to the need for him to become involved in the process of building a network of people who will support him in his good intentions (Manual, pp. 32-33). The value of building such a network is discussed only briefly in the manual because of the many differences among individual offending patterns and circumstances. Detailed discussion of network building is best left as the province of the therapist, who will need to consider the level of support and monitoring required for the individual offender, who should participate, and what special issues exist, especially those concerning family contact or reconstruction. Such questions are the focus of this section.

Experience suggests that although self-awareness and self-management are helpful in relapse prevention, sex abuse perpetrators need external controls as well. The experience of the Vermont Treatment Program for Sexual Aggressors indicates that perpetrators are not good at acknowledging lapse to therapists, and also that they neglect to employ their new skills in relapse prevention at critical moments. Pithers, Martin, and Cumming (1989) suggest that the internal, self-management dimension of relapse prevention does not prove adequate without an external, supervisory dimension. Pithers et al. see this supervisory dimension as serving three functions:

1. Enhancing the efficacy of probation or parole supervision by monitoring of specific offense precursors

2. Increasing the efficiency of supervision by creating an informed network of collateral contacts to assist the probation officer in monitoring the offender's behaviors

3. Creating a collaborative relationship between the probation officer and mental health professionals conducting therapy with the offender

Even in scenarios where the offender is no longer under the supervision of a probation officer, there are often a number of mental health or social work professionals engaged with the offender and/or his family. Collaborative relationships among those parties are crucial if the perpetrator is to be monitored effectively.

When to Start Building Networks

In line with the view that relapse prevention philosophy and planning should be an integral part of any therapy program, the development of networks should also be integral. If networking is to be effective, key people should be identified at the very beginning of any program. Usually at this stage they will be the key professionals who have referred the offender to the program and/or are working with his family. The early identification of key people enables them:

1. To be clear about the task: there is no cure. The aim of therapy is relapse prevention, and this will involve long term external monitoring as well as the development of internal controls by the perpetrator.
2. To attend regular reviews on the perpetrator as he moves through the program, to hear how he is progressing, and to comment on whether or not they can see positive change. This involvement makes them less vulnerable to manipulation by the perpetrator.

    In cases where key professionals are in touch with the perpetrator and/or his family while he is in therapy, they will be able to give crucial input on whether his behavior outside therapy is congruent with how he sounds in therapy sessions.
3. To develop an understanding of the pace of change and how realistic it is to consider family meetings, or in the longer term, family reconstruction, if this is an issue.

An offender who has done well in therapy and is at last being honest about his behavior often shows good self-knowledge in giving a detailed account of his offending pattern, sometimes admitting that he abused a child far more frequently than even the child describes. Clinical practice tells us that when a child is abused within a family context, the abuse has often taken place for years prior to disclosure. It is not unusual for a perpetrator to have committed thousands of separate offenses against one child for much of that child's life. In addition, research suggests that large numbers of men who abuse within families offend against extrafamilial children as well (Abel & Becker, 1987; Abel, Becker, Cunningham-Rathner, Mittelman, & Rouleau, 1988; Abel & Rouleau, 1990; Becker & Coleman, 1988; Faller, 1990; Weinrott & Saylor, 1991). When key child protection personnel are not involved until the very end of therapy, they may have to deal all at once with the fact that the perpetrator has a more established pattern of abuse than was originally thought, along with the fact that he has progressed well. This has the potential to create tensions and battles that could have been avoided had those personnel been involved from an earlier stage.

In some cases, it may be appropriate to involve other potentially key people from a very early stage, using the same rationale as described above. However, where family members are concerned, care should be taken not to involve them in isolation. They may need their own separate therapy. If they have had no therapy and the offender is still in an early stage of his own therapy, he may still try to manipulate, or groom, them. Nonabusing parents frequently have guilt and responsibility placed upon them by the offender, and may feel they must accept responsibility for ensuring that the offender does not reoffend. Monitoring and responsibility, however, are distinctly different.

Key people who should be involved at the earliest stages of the offender's therapy, in addition to the therapist responsible for that therapy, include (a) a named probation officer, psychiatrist, psychologist, or social worker, collaborating with (b) the named child sexual abuse specialist responsible for the child protection plan. It is crucial that at least one key person in the offender's network has the authority to take external action to control the offender or his environment.

When the Offender Has Abused Within His Family: Questions of Networking, Contact, and Family Reconstruction

When an offender has abused a child within his own family and wishes to return to that family, good networking is of paramount importance. The offender is likely to have manipulated all the family members in order that he could continue offending and maintain secrecy. It is crucial that the offender's therapist, child-care specialists and other network members, and the nonabusing partner work together in a way that places responsibility firmly on the offender and makes it more difficult for him to continue abusing family members and vulnerable children, regardless of whether or not family reconstruction is decided upon.

Work that involves family members may be valuable even if it is not aimed at family reconstruction. Family members may (a) be unsure what they want and need to do some work to find out; (b) want to check out what is possible; (c) never want to see the offender again, but are trying to make sense of family life in the environment he left behind; or (d) want to have contact with the offender but not want to live with him. Engaging in therapy in which key professionals work in an integrated way can help family members find out what they really want, so that they can make informed choices based on real information and knowledge about what the offender actually did and how he shifted blame and responsibility.

If family reconstruction is being considered, assessment of its viability needs to be the subject of ongoing therapy-based evaluation about what is and is not possible for a particular family. Early postdisclosure assessment, even if it is extensive, provides only a superficial understanding of what has happened. The amount of water under the bridge is revealed only in long-term work, hence any rash promises to family members about being "back together by Christmas" should be avoided. For example, early assessment interviews with Mark and his family presented him as a seductive abuser who used "gentle" tactics. Later admissions by Mark, as well as acting-out behaviors beginning to be exhibited by his young children, revealed him to be a sadistic offender who used a range of tactics to gain compliance but who particularly enjoyed seeing the children's pain.

Regardless of whether or not family reconstruction is a likely option, in cases where the offender is a father or stepfather, an important starting point for understanding family relationships is contained in the four preconditions for child sexual abuse identified by David Finkelhor (1984): (a) The offender is motivated to offend, (b) he overcomes his own internal inhibitors, (c) he overcomes external inhibitors, and (d) he overcomes the victim's resistance. Before family reconstruction can be considered, effective work should be done with each person in the context of these preconditions.

The offender's motivation to abuse must be addressed. This may be linked to a primary deviant arousal pattern and/or to other problems, such as revenge or anger motivation. His capacity for overcoming internal inhibitors to abuse must also be addressed. As Salter (1988) notes, "The internal inhibitions that should be present for offenders include empathy for the child and a rational appreciation of the harmfulness of the behavior. These are lacking in child sex offenders. . . . They show little true empathy for their victims and find it difficult to separate the point of view of the child from their own" (pp. 246-247). Clearly, the development of empathy and rational thinking is crucial if family reconstruction is to be considered, as is the existence of a relapse prevention plan built upon the offender's responsibility for his own actions. All of this takes time—there is no quick fix.

Parallel work must also take place with the nonabusing parent and extended family members, who the offender has overcome in the past through the use of manipulative tactics. Again, this work takes time. Work with the mother in particular should recognize that she has experienced trauma. Ovaris (1991) cites the grief cycle formulated by Elisabeth Kübler-Ross as a valuable model to use in understanding the mother's experience. The stages of this cycle are denial, anger, bargaining, depression, and acceptance. Ovaris notes that, "by understanding a mother's experience as a series of stages, the risk of either a 'helper' or mother getting stuck at one stage is reduced" (p. 19). Chaffin (1996) describes the mothers of child sexual abuse victims as

> individuals attempting to process a traumatic event, struggling to make sense of the abuse allegation for themselves and often benefiting from attention to their own needs for support, safety, and time to process the trauma. From a trauma processing perspective, features such as denial, unfocused anger, minimization of the problem, and ambivalence toward both the alleged victim and abuser would be considered par for the course, rather than evidence of toxic parenting or deep seated psychopathology. (p. 113)

Chaffin emphasizes the need to recognize the stages and steps that need to be taken, the first of which is to ensure that the mother is safe from ongoing trauma herself. Chaffin suggests that areas for work should include the mother's emotional needs, including a recognition that trauma needs to be processed, time should be allowed to make important decisions, and the importance of social supports and pressures should be recognized.

Our experience tells us that the mother in a family where child sexual abuse has taken place has many issues to address. The impact of the abuse on her as a woman should not be underestimated, even though the focus of intervention is often her role as partner or mother. She will be dealing with the sexual assault of her child and the ripple effect of the perpetrator's manipulative tactics on other relationships in the family including siblings and herself. She is likely to be hitting an all-time low. In the face of this, many competent and caring mothers can respond in ways not viewed as perfect by child protection professionals. Denial and disbelief are the most misunderstood responses of mothers. Such responses are often interpreted as supportive of the offender, whereas they may reflect the mother's need for survival and her wish for her child to have suffered less. One woman said, "If I believe what you're telling me, it means it really is that bad for my child. I don't want that for her." Shock, anger, distrust, powerlessness, confusion about sexual identity, fears for the future, and possible reawakening of personal survivor issues, on top of guilt and a sense of failure as a parent and a sexual partner, are some of the problems mothers tell us they experience.

Therapeutic work that takes place in the context of the offender and his partner meeting together needs to be handled with great care and due consideration to the likelihood of the offender attempting to manipulate his partner during the meeting itself. Understandably, the partner often wants to believe the abuse has not been that bad, and the offender may do all he can to reinforce that belief. Timing is of the essence; joint therapy sessions should be delayed until both the offender and the nonabusing partner have made sufficient progress in their individual therapy.

It is crucial to overlay whatever work is done with the mother of the abused child with knowledge of offenders, and of this specific offender, to help her see how the offender has manipulated her and her family. Wolf (1984) presents the notion of "groomed" environments. Post-disclosure, we often see a child victim who is closest to the offender and furthest away from everyone else in the family, especially the mother. This is no accident. Knowledge of offenders tells us that they arrange it that way. As one man said, "I drive a wedge between the child and anyone they might go to." Dysfunctional family dynamics don't cause sexual abuse; rather, sex offenders willfully exacerbate or create such dynamics. If family reconstruction or contact is being considered, the key purposes of therapy are to increase the mother's awareness and to empower her to take the necessary action to protect the children.

Parallel work must also be done with the child victims of sexual abuse whose resistance the offender has overcome in the past. In relation to this last precondition, it should be understood that the grooming tactics of many sex offenders are such that the victim may not physically resist, but rather may be subtly manipulated into pseudo-"consent" over a lengthy period of time.

Again, this work takes time and should not be rushed. The sequelae of abuse identified by Sgroi, Porter, and Blick (1982) may be present and need to be addressed in their own right. In addition, sexual abuse within a family is the corruption of an entire relationship, with a huge impact on the child's emotional, cognitive, and behavioral learning. Knowledge of offenders tells us that the child has probably been groomed to believe that he or she, not Daddy, is guilty and responsible. When an offender says, "It's something about you; you make me do it," that's a very powerful way of overcoming a child's resistance. Combined with "It'll kill your mother if she hears you've done this," it effectively prevents disclosure. It is often the best-groomed child who says, "I want my Daddy back; it wasn't his fault." Although children have a right to be heard, they also have the right not to become the mouthpiece of the offender.

Therapeutic work that involves meetings between the offender and the children he has abused should be approached with extreme care. Abuse does not start or stop with touch, and offenders may willfully or, in some cases, inadvertently say or do things that give hidden messages to children about continuing control. For example, an offender may have used the signal of a raised eyebrow to tell his daughter to go upstairs and await abuse. If later, in an apology meeting with his daughter, this offender says things that sound appropriate, but raises an eyebrow while doing so, he may push her into a flashback to the abuse, and she may go into all the feelings she had at the time. She may feel as powerless in that meeting as she did at the time she was being abused. The fact that this is happening secretly and in front of those who are supposed to be protecting her compounds her suffering. In earlier work, we have described the need for careful ground rules for apology meetings with adult survivors (Eldridge & Still, 1995). Where children are concerned, yet more safeguards are necessary, and timing should take account of the stage each party has reached in his or her own therapy.

Grooming needs to be fully revealed in order for the family to be reconstructed in a new way in which children can be heard and believed and the offender cannot operate undetected. This includes work with any siblings who have been groomed and whose resistance might be overcome by the offender in the future.

The following are questions the therapist should ask when considering family contact for an offender or family reconstruction. If either is to be entertained, all of these questions should be answered in the affirmative.

Regarding the Offender's Progress

- Has the offender accepted full responsibility for his targeting, grooming, and offending behaviors?
- Has the offender developed empathy for his victim(s)?
- Has the offender accepted that the needs of the children are paramount?
- Is there scope for secure, nonabusive attachment between the offender and the child(ren) he abused?
- Is there scope for secure, nonabusive attachment between the offender and any children who were not directly abused?
- Has the offender worked out effective ways of modifying/controlling his sexuality in the future?
- Has the offender developed a primarily internal as opposed to external attributional style?
- Does the offender have a positive attitude toward change?
- Does the offender have a clear understanding of his offending cycle?
- Has the offender worked out a realistic relapse prevention plan that enlists the help of other people without relying on them?
- Is the offender's behavior congruent with what he says?
- Is the offender's long-term prognosis for change positive?
- Does the offender have a noncollusive support network comprising the following kinds of people? (a) nonabusing partner, (b) named adult family member(s) with authority, (c) named adults outside the family with authority, (d) named adult friends, (e) named adults having authority within the local community (e.g., minister, doctor, teacher), (f) named sex offender therapist (e.g., probation officer, psychiatrist, psychologist, social worker) collaborating with the named child sexual abuse specialist responsible for the child protection plan

Regarding the Offender and the Nonabusing Partner in Relationship

- Is there a positive relationship between the nonabusing and abusing parents (e.g., in terms of equality, lack of collusion, good communication)?
- Has the nonabusing partner become the primary power base within the family in relation to the children? (Is this real authority, or just increased responsibility without power?)
- While recognizing that the offender is responsible for offending, is the nonabusing partner willing to accept the role of external inhibitor in the future?
- Does the partner know as much as is appropriate about the offender's cycle? That is, does she know what signs to be alert for?
- Does the partner know as much as is appropriate about the offender's relapse prevention plan?
- Does the partner feel able to challenge the offender without fear of reprisal?
- Does the partner know which other children are most at risk of being targeted by the offender? Does she have adequate plans for managing this risk?

Regarding the Nonabusing Partner

- Does the nonabusing partner really want family reconstruction, or is she just saying so to please or pacify someone else?
- Have the nonabusing partner's own key issues been addressed in therapy?
- Does the partner now have insight into how she was previously disempowered/manipulated by the offender?
- Has the partner accepted that the needs of the children are paramount?
- Does the partner show no signs of scapegoating or blaming the victim(s)?
- Is there scope for secure attachment between the nonabusing partner and the child(ren) the offender abused?
- Is there scope for secure attachment between the nonabusing partner and any children who were not directly abused?
- Does the partner have another adult within the family to turn to should she be concerned that the offender is heading into his cycle?

- Does the partner have another adult outside the family to turn to should she be concerned that the offender is heading into his cycle?
- Does the partner have a professional to turn to should she be concerned that the offender is heading into his cycle?

Regarding the Child Who Has Been Sexually Abused

- Does the child want family reconstruction?
- Is family reconstruction in the child's interests?
- Have the child's key issues been addressed in his or her therapy?
- Does the child really want the offender back even after he or she has become free of the offender's grooming tactics?
- Does the child truly recognize that the offender was solely responsible for the abuse?
- Have the child and those close to him or her worked out a language for or method by which the child can communicate anxieties in the future? (These should relate not only to the offender's behavior but to his moods and very presence as well—anything that makes the child feel uncomfortable. The child may experience affective flashbacks. These should be taken seriously in their own right, but they may also be a possible intuitive recognition by the child of a precursor to further offending.)
- Does the child feel close to the nonoffending parent and feel that he or she can turn to that parent and be protected if the child feels uncomfortable about the offender?
- Does the child have another adult within the extended family to whom he or she can turn and be protected if he or she feels uncomfortable about the offender?
- Does the child have another adult outside the family to whom he or she can turn and be protected if he or she feels uncomfortable about the offender? (Such a person should be an official member of the family's child protection network—for example, a designated teacher.)
- Does the child have a social worker to whom he or she can turn and be protected if he or she feels uncomfortable about the offender?

Regarding Siblings of the Child Who Has Been Sexually Abused

Appropriate questions regarding siblings would include all those listed above regarding the child victim, as well as the following:

- Do the siblings understand the effects of sexual abuse on the victim?
- Are the siblings supportive of the victim?

Regarding the Family

- Do adults and children recognize that the offender is responsible for the abuse?
- Do authority figures within the extended family have a clear understanding that the offender is responsible for the abuse?
- Do adults and children understand the effects of the sexual abuse on the victim(s)?
- Are authority figures within the extended family supportive of the children and the nonabusing partner?
- Have all members of the family accepted that the needs of the children are paramount?
- Has work been done with dyads and triads within the family as appropriate?
- Has there been appropriate therapy for all members of the family who have been affected?
- Have the family members been able to positively change the family dynamics the offender created or exploited in order to facilitate abuse?
- Are there sufficient professional resources available to work with family members before and after the offender's possible return?
- Does the family have a positive attitude toward professional intervention? (For example, can family members work in therapy without becoming hostile or overly dependent?)
- Do family members know as much as is appropriate for them to know about the offender's cycle and relapse prevention plan?
- Does everyone in the family understand why the offender is not allowed to do certain things, such as perform certain child-care tasks or be alone with young children?
- Do adult family members recognize which children within the extended family might be most at risk from the offender? Do they have adequate plans for managing this risk?
- Is there an acceptable level of consensus that facilitates all the above?

Conclusion

All of the parties concerned may engage in therapy, but still may never reach a point where family reconstruction can be considered a safe option. It must be emphasized that the questions listed above as guidelines assume ongoing assessment of the offender's progress in developing and implementing a realistic relapse prevention plan, thereby facilitating the protection of children from physical/sexual abuse. The question of who really wants family reconstruction—the victim, the nonabusing parent, the siblings, the offender—must be considered continuously.

Also a necessity is ongoing assessment of (a) how these considerations are then processed by family members, individually and collectively; (b) what other kinds of risk exist (e.g., not only of physical sexual abuse and ill treatment but of other forms of "significant harm," through impairment of health or development); and (c) whether continuing agency, community, family support, and monitoring are available.

Phase 2

From the Midpoint of Therapy Onward

The material included in this section is linked to the Phase 2 material in *Maintaining Change: A Personal Relapse Prevention Manual* (Manual, pp. 35-152), which focuses on three key areas:

- *Section A:* This part of the manual is concerned with the offender's thinking, feeling, and behavioral cycles and the identification of linked routes to relapse, key risk patterns, and the development of strategies to deal with lapse.
- *Section B:* This section addresses the offender's need to prevent and deal with risky moods through the use of exercises designed to help him change his thought and feeling patterns. There is an emphasis on changing feelings through the changing of negative thinking patterns. The focus is on generalized distortions rather than on offense-specific distortions.
- *Section C:* This section is intended to help the offender develop a personal relapse prevention collection that includes both internal and external monitoring.

The therapist can hand the material in Phase 2 out to the offender in sections or en bloc. Feedback from offenders about what works best for them suggests that individuals have very different views. Some like to work on all three sections at once, whereas others feel overwhelmed by this approach and prefer to take the material step by step. Hence, it is best for the therapist to ask each offender which approach he would prefer.

The continued building of support and monitoring networks is also discussed in this phase, both in this guide and in the personal relapse prevention manual.

Personal Relapse Prevention Manual, Phase 2, Section A: The Cycle and Routes to Relapse

The exercises in Phase 2, Section A of the manual (Manual, pp. 35-75) are designed to help the offender use his developing awareness of his offending pattern to recognize early danger signals, take avoiding action, and thereby prevent reoffending. The exercise titled "Alert List for Cycle" (Manual, pp. 36-53) focuses on thoughts, moods, and behaviors at different points in the offender's cycle. Handouts and exercises that deal with lapse and relapse help the offender to recognize lapses, especially in the context of risky scenarios, and begin making plans to cope with them. Common routes to relapse, which can include many different lapse scenarios, are identified. The handouts provide examples of offenders who have taken these routes and the ways they have coped, or failed to cope. Such examples provide a nonthreatening vehicle for introducing offenders to concepts to which they can relate. The notion of fictional characters following routes to relapse helps people think, "Yes, I might just do that," or "Yes, that's like what I did—and if that guy could take avoiding action, maybe I could too!"

Self-monitoring of thoughts, feelings, and behaviors is introduced, and monitoring sheets are provided. These are designed to increase the likelihood of their being completed accurately. Many offenders worry about completing diary-type tasks because they fear that their work might fall into the wrong hands. Thus the "Urge to Lapse Monitoring Sheet" (Manual, p. 72) and the "Lapse Monitoring Sheet" (Manual, p. 73) have space available for the offender to record time, place, mood, thoughts, and coping skills used, but no space allotted for details of who was there and exactly what took place. These details are for the offender to discuss with the therapist.

As soon as the offender reaches a point in therapy where he becomes concerned with developing an offense-free life, the therapist may introduce him to some of the concepts associated with relapse prevention. These are included in the manual in handout form and are described below.

Lapse and Relapse

The offender needs to learn that lapse and relapse are different, that lapses are likely, and that he need not be overwhelmed by a lapse. *Relapsing* can be defined as reoffending in any form. *Lapsing* is taking one of the steps previously noted as one that leads toward reoffending, such as watching children and spending time fantasizing about them sexually. Thoughts that "flit" across the mind must be expected; these don't constitute lapse unless the offender allows them to become persistent. Lapse may take the form of several stages of increasing riskiness along the road to relapse. Whether or not relapse takes place will depend on how the offender deals with lapse.

Main Routes to Relapse

The offender needs to learn the most common routes to relapse as well as those that are his own most likely routes. Four common routes are:

- unexpected risky scenarios;
- a perpetrator's testing himself out;
- an overload of offense-related sights, sounds, and moods; and
- development of a high-risk state of mind.

Each of these routes is discussed in turn below (see Figure 3).

As part of the discussion of lapse and routes to relapse, the term *scenario* is introduced in the personal relapse prevention manual (Manual, p. 56) as follows:

> Lapses do not result only from physical situations. They involve combinations of a person's thoughts, feelings, and behaviors in relation to other people and events. In other words, each situation is a bit like a script for a scene in a play or film: a scenario. This is real life, though, and you are in control of the part your own character plays. You write your own script for the real-life scene. The word *scenario* is used throughout this manual to refer to the coming together of your thoughts, feelings, and behaviors with other people and events. Always remember that you play a key part in determining the course of events!

Unexpected Risky Scenarios

During therapy, an offender may say that he intends to avoid children completely in the future. Although it is possible for him to ensure that he does not volunteer for child-care activities and plan to avoid being alone with children, it will be impossible for him to avoid children altogether. The world is full of children. High-risk scenarios may arise that are not of his own making; for example, a child may be lost in the street or supermarket and approach him, or a child may ask him how to work a vending machine. A friend may invite him for a meal and

58

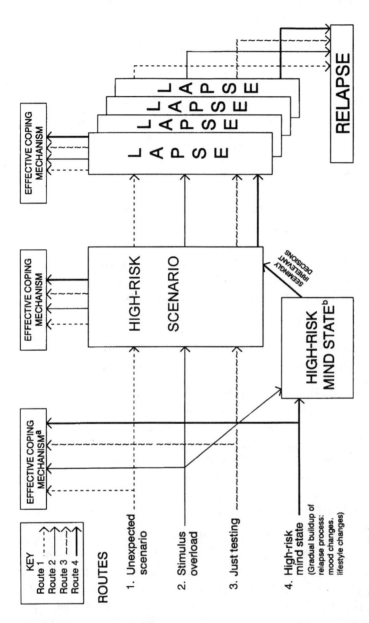

Figure 3. Routes to Relapse

a. Early recognition of a route can allow an offender to avoid a high-risk scenario, provided he invokes effective coping mechanisms.
b. At this point, the offender is likely to make seemingly irrelevant decisions that can lead to lapse and thus to relapse; he needs external network support.

children may call at the house. The offender needs to have flexible plans for dealing with the unexpected.

Offenders' definitions of unexpected events are sometimes worth challenging. They are often highly predictable rather than unexpected and may link with seemingly irrelevant or unimportant decisions. For example, everyone except an offender would realize that children might still be in the changing room at a public pool just prior to the adults' time to swim. The unexpected events mentioned by an offender may be likely only in the world of the sex offender, and may suggest that he behaves in ways that make such events likely. For example, how many strange children approach you in supermarkets?

"Just Testing"

Offenders sometimes want to test out their self-control by putting themselves into risky scenarios. A fixated pedophile who has made a career out of abusing children may start by allowing himself to be around children in the company of others. If he feels in control of himself, he may then allow himself to baby-sit while the child's parents go out. Next, he might allow himself to bathe the child, just to show how much in control he really is. This is similar to someone who has had a massive drinking problem allowing himself to go into bars, and then to have liquor in his home—only to look at, of course!

An offending father who has been allowed to return to his family because his presence appears to be a manageable risk within the context of a carefully thought-out child protection plan may begin to erode the plan by testing himself in different scenarios. He might think, for example, "I feel in control, so I could just test to see if I can put the children to bed without touching them sexually."

The "just testing" rationale is worth questioning. It may simply be that the offender is deluding himself in order to avoid admitting to himself that he is planning to reoffend, or he may believe that this is a respectable rationale to put forward to his therapist. In process terms, one "just testing" act can lead to more and more risky behaviors.

Overload of Offense-Related Sights, Sounds, and Moods

Most offending cycles involve not just thoughts and behavior, but senses and moods. For example, an offender who was particularly attracted to fair-haired 10-year-old boys, and who has regularly targeted such boys in public swimming pools, may enter a therapy program and make good progress in changing his thinking and arousal pattern. However, one day after his therapy has ended, he may be walking down the street feeling quite depressed and in need of comfort. Suddenly, walking toward him he sees a small, fair-haired boy. Nearby, someone is washing a shop floor with a chlorine-based cleaner, and from another shop he hears some music that was popular during a phase of his offending that he found particularly enjoyable.

If this offender has no means of identifying and dealing with these stimuli, he may experience a very strong urge to fantasize about reoffending. He may feel that this is an overpowering force that has come from nowhere, and that he has no control over it. The speed with which the stimuli come together may seem to him to be so fast that he lacks the time to bring to bear antioffending devices that he may have as yet only partially internalized. Hence it is very important that offenders in therapy identify their mood and senses cycles and plan how to deal with offense-related stimuli in order to maintain offense-free lives.

High-Risk Mind-State (Mood) Route to Relapse

This is the development of a high risk state of mind already known to be associated with reoffending (in the case of inhibited cycles) or likely to become so post-intervention (in the case of continuous cycles).

Before intervention, offenders with continuous cycles may have been as likely to say, "I'm feeling great today; this would be a good day to go out and find some boys" as to say, "I'm feeling low; some boys would cheer me up!" After successful intervention, armed with newly inhibited cycles, these offenders may still feel there's something missing on good days, but may find replacing this with non-abusive behaviors easier on good days than on bad days. Everyone feels low sometimes and this is when negative thinking can be used to create full blown bad days. Offenders who have high levels of emotional loneliness and poor self-esteem are particularly susceptible, especially if offending has been central to their lives and they haven't found adequate replacements. Offenders whose cycles were inhibited prior to intervention may remain susceptible to the patterns of thinking, feeling, and behaving they used to overcome internal inhibitors in the past.

Negative emotion can lead through a series of lapses that, when dealt with negatively, progress to relapse. Cummings, Gordon, and Marlatt (1980) have noted the role of negative emotional states in precipitating relapse across the addictions. This is a particularly dangerous route that may lead quickly from lapse to relapse if uninterrupted. Pithers, Marques, Gibat, and Marlatt (1983) describe the relapse process as beginning with emotional susceptibility and progressing through fantasy and cognitive distortion to planning and then acting. Offenders whose cycles are sometimes inhibited and who need an excuse to reoffend are susceptible to this route to relapse. Pithers et al. suggest that offenders should learn to identify their risk factors and the cues that can alert them to the existence of each risk factor, and then develop coping strategies to deal with each cue. This strategy is particularly useful in relation to the high-risk mood route to relapse.

The development of a high-risk mind state can work as follows: The offender may have generalized cognitive distortions (e.g., unrealistic expectations) about himself and other people, a tendency to see himself as a failure if he doesn't fill his life with "shoulds" and duties, leaving himself very little time for enjoyable "wants." In the term used by G. Alan Marlatt (1989a, 1989b), the offender develops a "lifestyle imbalance."

Neil, a church minister with a strongly inhibited cycle, made the following comments:

> It's a question of persuading yourself after each abusive incident that you can stop the abuse. It was as if I knew that God would be angry with me but he'd understand and if I worked hard enough after the offenses he would forgive me and decide that it was better to forgive than to lose the good work I was achieving.
>
> The promise to never do it again would last for some months, but it was a negative spiral, because I was guilt-ridden after each offense and promised myself this would have to stop. I almost tried to purge my offenses by working even harder than I'd worked before, thinking this would occupy me and would get rid of whatever sexual pressures were present. What I actually did was by working harder and for the wrong reasons, I felt I was not achieving as I should, not doing my job properly. It caused enormous stress that I hadn't coped with.

Neil then "coped" with the stress by using what he knew would make him feel better quickly: masturbation linked to fantasies of abuse. He became increasingly obsessed with the fantasies, which included permission-giving distorted thinking, and before long he began planning and abusing again. Post-intervention monitoring of an offender like Neil would involve checking on his lifestyle, his workload, and his expectations of himself.

In the author's experience, many offenders with such a pattern are also inclined toward automatic negative thinking. This works as follows: the offender homes in on the negative aspect of any scenario, tending to see one small mistake as total failure. This leads to a feeling of being a failure in all things, unfairly treated, cheated, and deprived. The bad feeling grows, reducing the offender's capacity for positive thinking further and further, until he can see nothing positive. One might imagine someone blowing up a balloon until all he can see in front of him is the balloon. The "bad feeling balloon" becomes all.

The bad feeling or emotion makes the offender want to escape, but positive means of escape or coping are blocked along with positive thought. Hence there is a tendency for him to seek escape through avenues that have comforted him in the past—that is, where there are positive expectations about indulging in the behavior as a rapid mood changer—even though these avenues have caused long-term problems in the past. At this point, the offender chooses short-term immediate gratification over long-term delayed negative consequences. Marlatt (1989a, 1989b) describes this most aptly as "choosing to feed the PIG [problem of immediate gratification]." The offender begins to fantasize in order to hide his bad feeling balloon behind another that will block it.

In this connection, it is important to remember that although in therapy, offenders need to recognize the harm they've done, and may experience some level of depression when they allow themselves to do so, they should not be encouraged to remain in this phase of change for so long that they begin needing to escape the bad feeling and thereby feed the cycle by returning to comforting old fantasies which legitimate their behavior.

When an offender begins seeking comfort in fantasies, he may return to fantasies in which he has sought comfort in the past—namely, about children he has abused. In his fantasies, he may imagine the children smiling, enjoying it, consenting. He has to believe this in order to feel better, which is the object of the exercise. In the terms offenders have used to describe this process, "It's like putting a mask of our choosing on the child's face. The mask covers the child's real expression and prevents us from having to see this." An offender who is motivated primarily by revenge or anger may indulge in fantasies in which other people's behavior gives him the right to cause suffering. This also requires self-delusion and distorted thinking.

At times, however, whiffs of reality may break through the offender's distorted thinking. These in turn create guilt feelings and blow up the balloon of bad feelings even more. In order to combat this, he must further blow up his fantasy/distorted thinking balloon, thus leading to a refusal to recognize any harm, and to even greater distortions. If he allows himself to believe that what he fantasizes about doing is okay, then why not carry it out? Why not think about actually doing it again, because it won't do any harm? Hence the move from fantasy through increasingly distorted thinking into planning and, eventually, action.

Offenders with this pattern are often enabled to talk about it just by being shown a chart with the words: *Emotion, Fantasy, Distorted Thinking, Planning,* and *Action,* and being asked "Does this mean anything to you?" Ralph, a multiple abuser of extrafamilial children, responded to such a question by saying:

The emotion can be more or less anything. Feeling down, feeling things aren't going right, receiving bad news, feelings of loss, not being able to see my family. The emotion I don't want to deal with, I don't want to deal with the feelings. I want to get rid of them and I know an easy way of getting rid of them is to go into fantasy. Fantasies of being with a child and being sexual with a child. The way to get rid of the emotions is that the child wants to be with me as well—that it's mutual. That we're both enjoying it. It gets rid of all the emotions.

And the fantasy itself backs up all the distorted thinking, which is that children do like having sex with me and that they enjoy my company, that they want to do this as much as me, that I'm not hurting them, and I back all that up again with fantasy about my childhood, using images of me being abused, which has been finely cut down—I've edited out all the times they did hurt me, so all I've got is the abuse that I thought was okay that I saw as not hurting me, and I can use that in connection with fantasies of children. Also using reality as well, setting up times to be alone with the child but actually turning it around and saying it's the child that wants to be with me, that they like it because they're always with me, when in fact it's me that's setting that situation up.

The fantasy actually becomes planning for me. I plan everything in fantasy. I plan which children I can be around, I even work out what could go wrong and how I could get around that, and deal with that. Once I'm running fantasies and planning, it then becomes like there's no choice. Once I'm alone with a child I've got to do this, I can't do anything else, there's no other way of getting rid of the feelings. So I've gone from feeling lost, feeling angry, basically then moving right through to the stage of abusing a child, merely because I felt lonely or things weren't going my way.

I can knock anything into the emotions, and it's just a matter of time once I start using fantasy unless I do something to stop that. Then the fantasy itself becomes in a sense self-propelling: The more I fantasize, the more I need to fantasize, to make the fact I'm fantasizing okay. I need to keep doing it to make it okay to stop the guilt coming in, and the other emotions coming back, which again self-propels the distorted thinking. Everything becomes okay again, the planning increases, I lose sight of obvious things. I don't take notice of how much time I'm spending with children, then it's back into the action again of actually abusing.

Ralph has a much faster operating cycle than Neil, the church minister quoted above, and once he is in a high-risk mood, his risk of reoffending is imminent. Ralph needs a relapse prevention plan that reflects the speed of his cycle, with an emphasis on prevention of emotional buildup, specific work related to his own victim experiences, and external monitoring.

An offender who has allowed himself to reach a high-risk mind state probably needs outside network support and intervention. Many offenders talk about this state as a feeling that they are in a bubble, isolated from the world. An offender in such a bubble is unlikely to be able to deal with high-risk scenarios without lapsing, and may indulge in a series of seemingly irrelevant decisions leading to the opportunity to reoffend. For example, an offender may start being late for work and may get into arguments with his boss about it. One day, after he's given a final warning, he just happens to realize he's going to be late again. He just happens to think that if he takes a shortcut through the park, past the children's playground, he'll be on time. As he passes the play area, he looks at his watch and realizes he's missed the bus anyway. He hasn't had any breakfast, it's a nice day, so he'll buy a meal at the café in the park, which he just happens to be passing. He sits down in the café, in which all the tables just happen to overlook the children's play area. And so on and so on.

If an offender in a high-risk mind state comes across an unexpected high-risk scenario, he is likely to regard this as a golden opportunity to offend, an intervention of fate. He will already be seeking excuses to reoffend. He may well plan to put himself into high-risk scenarios, simply in order to be able to act.

Effective Coping Mechanisms to
Deal With High-Risk Scenarios

The offender needs to learn detailed effective coping mechanisms related to high-risk scenarios that can lead to lapse. For example, if he has an inhibited cycle and needs to provide himself with an excuse to offend, he may be particularly inclined toward the development of a high-risk mind state. Hence he will need to make major lifestyle changes and work on replacing automatic negative thinking with positive thinking. He will also need to plan how to maintain that position, and how to deal with times when he faces problems and his hopes are not being realized. He needs to develop a range of coping mechanisms that work for him.

As has already been noted, there are other routes to high-risk scenarios, and hence an offender who is not in a high-risk mind state may reach them via those different routes. However, his response to the high-risk scenario may be (a) to take appropriate avoiding action by implementing previously learned effective coping mechanisms to deal with high-risk scenarios, or (b) to lapse, if he has no such mechanisms and/or is an automatic negative thinker who sees minor errors or occasional thoughts of offending as a sign of total failure. The first response not only leads away from lapse but also increases self-confidence and feelings of self-efficacy, thus decreasing the general risk of reoffending every time it is used successfully. The second response, on the other hand, may lead in the opposite direction (see Figure 4).

Effective Coping Mechanisms to Deal With Lapse

If the offender does lapse—that is, takes one of the steps leading toward reoffending—the route he takes thereafter may depend on how far he is along the road to developing a high-risk mind state. If this is not in place, the chosen route may depend on whether he has learned effective coping mechanisms to deal with lapse and/or whether he is an automatic negative thinker who tends to see one small error as a major failure.

If, for example, the offender has lapsed by allowing himself to masturbate on one occasion while thinking about offending, he can deal with that by recognizing the dangers this act presents and, instead of

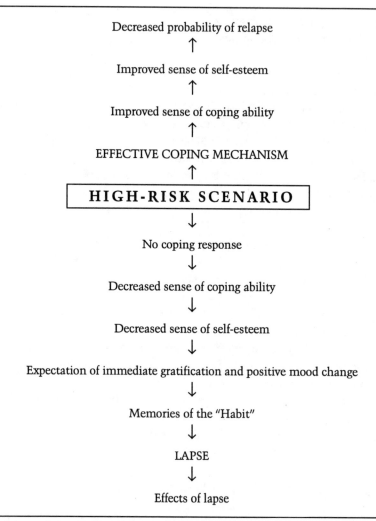

Decreased probability of relapse
↑
Improved sense of self-esteem
↑
Improved sense of coping ability
↑
EFFECTIVE COPING MECHANISM
↑

HIGH-RISK SCENARIO

↓
No coping response
↓
Decreased sense of coping ability
↓
Decreased sense of self-esteem
↓
Expectation of immediate gratification and positive mood change
↓
Memories of the "Habit"
↓
LAPSE
↓
Effects of lapse

Figure 4. Responses to High-Risk Scenarios

being afraid of it or feeling that he has failed, taking appropriate action—namely, employing a previously learned effective coping mechanism to prevent a further lapse. When the offender uses a coping mechanism successfully, this increases his self-confidence and sense of being in control. He effectively empowers himself in relation to the problem, and a side benefit can be that he begins to feel more in control of his life generally (see Figure 5).

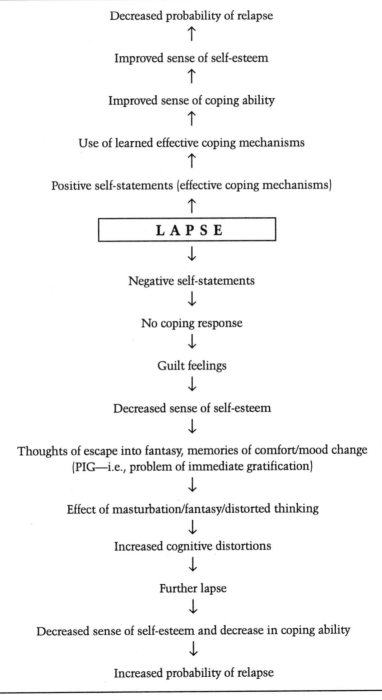

Figure 5. Responses to Lapse

Preventing Relapse: A Summary

In preventing relapse, the offender must take responsibility for:

1. Identifying and understanding his own pattern in detail.
2. Taking a positive, realistic attitude toward everyday life.
3. Developing a rewarding offense-free lifestyle in which the emotional needs he met by offending are dealt with or met in positive ways.
4. Developing a self-image that does not fit with offending.
5. Finding mechanisms—which work fast!—for countering automatic negative thoughts before they create a feeling that blocks out all positive rational thoughts and good feelings about self-worth.
6. Anticipating high-risk scenarios, and planning how to avoid them if possible, and how to deal with them should they occur, by the use of effective coping mechanisms.
7. Ensuring that the relapse prevention plan is live, active, and at his fingertips. He should be able to demonstrate this by acting out key scenarios, being able to give immediate answers to "What will you do if . . . " questions and follow-up questions (e.g., "And if it doesn't go as planned, and [a particular high-risk scenario] happens unexpectedly—what will you do?"). Action is often more effective than sitting and thinking. If the scenario is really risky, the offender needs to (a) recognize it as such and (b) get out and keep out.
8. Distinguishing between lapse and relapse and planning how to avoid and deal with lapse if it occurs, by using effective coping mechanisms.
9. Keeping regular contact with members of his designated external monitoring network. This includes keeping call back appointments with therapists from his therapy program who helped him design his relapse prevention plan.

Personal Relapse Prevention Manual, Phase 2, Section B: Preventing and Dealing With Risky Moods

In Section B of Phase 2 in the personal relapse prevention manual (Manual, pp. 77-123), the offender is introduced to a multipronged attack on the buildup of risky moods. This includes making changes in behavior and thinking patterns and working on ways of dealing with stress, if it is still experienced.

The development of risky mood states plays a major part in increasing the risk of reoffending, even for offenders who have responded well in their programs. The offender is introduced to this in the manual in a way that takes account of the possibility of both continuous and inhibited cycles and uses comments about ordinary human processes to which he can relate. The introduction to this section in the personal relapse prevention manual (Manual, p. 77) states:

> You may know all about the power of risky moods based on your understanding of your past offending pattern. However, you may be someone who wasn't trying to stop offending in the past and who offended regardless of what mood you were in. Now that you are involved in a therapy program, you've learned many good reasons for giving up offending. You've developed some internal inhibitors—that is, some internal stops that say, "I must not do this." You'll probably find, like most people who try to give up something they've enjoyed, that it's when you're in certain moods that you're most likely to say "To hell with it" and get past your internal stops.

Offenders who have never tried to give up sex offending may have tried to give up or cut down on something else, such as smoking, eating, gambling, or drinking. From these experiences, they should be able to relate to the concept of feeling low and seeking comfort in activities they know will make them feel better quickly—namely, the thing they were supposed to be giving up.

The handout titled "The Risky Mood Relapse Process: At-a-Glance Guide" (Manual, p. 78) introduces the offender to the way positive thinking can be used to break into the relapse process from its earliest stage. Examples of effective coping strategies to deal with each stage of this process are suggested. The offender is given an exercise sheet to write down what he thinks will work for him.

Lifestyle Imbalance

The concept of lifestyle imbalance is the rationale for the exercises concerned with changing lifestyle and developing a personally satisfying offense-free lifestyle (Manual, pp. 85-97). The emphasis is on safe, nonabusive "wants," rather than on virtuous "shoulds." Wants may be unrealistic, hence the offender is encouraged to look at what he has achieved in the past, what realistic new ideas he can add, and how he can plan for the future. Steps on the way to achievement are emphasized.

Mark has described feeling as if he's in a bubble, insulated from the world, in the lead-up to his offending. The following dialogue shows how Mark is beginning to make links between feeling states and unrealistic dreams:

Therapist: What do you know about yourself going into a bad feeling state?

Mark: Having fantasies about abusing children under people's noses and not being caught is one sign, so I use positive fantasy instead. I'd imagine being successful in the job I want.

Therapist: But suppose those were unrealistic fantasies; how would that work?

Mark: It could cause me to be too sure of myself and have a bad attitude to people.

Therapist: Where would that lead?

Mark: To being abusive to them, being aggressive, that would put me back into a "couldn't care less" attitude, lead me back into PIG, lead me back into "look after number one" mode. There's looking after your own needs, but there's a "looking after number one" state I've been in many times before. I go into it, and to hell with everybody and everything else.

Therapist: Sometimes you can get hooked on unrealistic fantasies and then disappointed because they don't come true?

Mark: Yes, I've done that, but then my "self-talk" says, "But you know that's not possible now, and not at the speed you want it. May take another few years, or may not get to it. Don't run, slow down, takes time, get your patience back."

Therapist: Is that a sign of trouble, if you're losing patience?

Mark: Yes, it goes into the nasty self-preservation mode. There's so many links. I try to take a laid-back approach and try and look at it from the outside. I'm going to keep a journal of thoughts and how I dealt with them.

Many habitual offenders have spent so much time building their lives around offending that they don't have many ideas about what to do in an offense-free life. One way they might begin is by collecting information, and the manual suggests some places where they might start to do this. These suggestions will work most safely if the therapist helps modify the offender's plans, using application of local knowledge. Some of the local resources listed in the manual may appear to be okay for the offender to contact, but they may be problematic in practice. The manual also encourages the offender to keep a calendar on which to plan interesting nonabusive things to do.

The buildup of high levels of stress is often described by offenders as a precursor to reoffending after breaks in their cycle. Knowing how to relax physically can help an offender overcome such stress, hence a relaxation exercise is included in the manual (Manual, pp. 98-101).

Changing Negative Thinking Patterns

One of the main ways in which risky moods develop is through negative thinking. Hence it is crucial for offenders to learn to change their feelings by changing their thinking patterns. The exercises included in the manual to combat negative thinking are adapted from the ideas of Aaron Beck (1976) and David Burns (1981). The introduction to these exercises (Manual, p. 102) presents them in a way offenders can relate to:

> The thoughts you have affect the way you feel. You know that thinking about offending in fantasy makes you want to do it more and makes it feel more okay to do it. Similarly, the thoughts you have about yourself and other people affect how you feel about yourself and about them. If you get into depressed moods before offending, it is worth your while to do the following exercises to see if the way you think generally makes you more likely to feel miserable and low. It's not just thoughts about sex offending that lead to offending; thoughts that make you feel worthless, sad, lonely, rejected, and angry can also make you feel you've got an excuse to offend.
>
> These thoughts are not always rational—that is, they are not always based on what has really happened. They're often based on the worst possible view of what has happened. If you're a negative thinker, you're probably inclined to focus on what went wrong in any scenario, rather than on what went right. For example, when you look back on a day at work, you remember the problems you had rather than what went well—and you begin to feel depressed. Someone who thinks positively will recognize what went wrong, but will focus on what went well and how to build on that.
>
> You can change the way you think. If you're a negative thinker, remember that you were not born that way; it has just become a habit with you—a habit you can change!

The concepts of automatic thoughts (i.e., instant responses to what happens), common types of generalized thinking error, and ways of challenging these, as described by David Burns, are highly user-friendly. I have adapted these concepts to address the kind of thoughts and thinking patterns most often described to me by sex offenders as linked to their relapse process. It is useful to work through the types of thinking error with each person to ensure that they are clearly understood. If group members identify new types that have meaning for them, then adopt them.

"Finding the Source of Your Thinking"

The exercise "Finding the Source of Your Thinking" (Manual, pp. 113-115) is a valuable addition to relapse prevention collections for regular use. Offenders are asked to use it when they have a negative thought. They are asked to write down the thought and then ask, "What would it mean if that were true?" They write that down. They ask again, what would it mean to me if that second comment was true. They continue until they think they've reached their main concern. Some people move through many thoughts and interpretations in doing this exercise; others finish very quickly. For example, Sam thought, "John and Sue don't like me"; that means "I can't get along with adults"; that means "Only children like me"; that means "They're attracted to me too"; that means "It'll be okay to have sex with that little boy at the swimming club who smiled at me!" Vince, on the other hand, eventually reached the same place, but went through three pages of thoughts and meanings first.

After completing this exercise, the offender is asked to return to the beginning of the chain and challenge the logic of each thought in turn. Much of this thinking is linked to excuses to offend, and if the offender catches it early, he can challenge both his generalized and his offense-related thinking errors.

Thoughts and Feelings

Failure to recognize feelings and fear of feelings are not uncommon among sex offenders and can be linked to buildup of stress and a sense of being a victim in an unfair world. Jim, an emotionally lonely man, said: "Part of having a positive way of life is living with feelings. I used to switch myself off from feelings unless they were happy ones. I would just say, 'I don't feel anything.' I wouldn't let myself feel any hurt, nor let people see. I might be dying inside really, but I'd just shrug my shoulders."

Nick abused children through his role as a trusted family friend who was always there to help out. Even in his intervention program, Nick always had to be Mr. Nice Guy, and even under extreme provocation would smile and say, "Yes, that's fine." This pattern may have developed when he was a child being abused by adults, but it had become habitual. The following dialogue shows how Nick is beginning to use emotion recognition skills and positive rational thinking in combination.

> *Nick:* If I have a really strong feeling of anger and I continually suppress it, it's seething and boiling, I take it out in a manipulative, abusive way, that puts me on what I think is an even keel, but actually everyone's hurt, including me. What I'm trying to do now is allow myself to recognize the feeling, feel it, pause, think, and then act. That stops me from both repressing and exploding. I've a fear of how adults perceive me. I don't want to be seen as an angry person. If I give vent to my feelings, that would lead people to see me as aggressive.
>
> *Therapist:* What would it mean to you if that were true?
>
> *Nick:* If I was seen as aggressive, people would talk behind my back.
>
> *Therapist:* And that would mean?
>
> *Nick:* If people talk about me they would no longer want to talk to me.
>
> *Therapist:* That's how you think, but do you believe all that's true?
>
> *Nick:* [Using his "Finding the Source of Your Thinking" exercise] No, going back to the first thought, the rational argument would be that people wouldn't see me as aggressive just because I expressed my feelings, provided, of course, that I expressed it in an okay way. The rational argument against people talking behind my back would be, "Even if one does, they wouldn't all do that, and some would say I'd changed for the better, that I was showing my feelings a bit more." As for the next fear, well it's not true at all that because someone talks about you they don't want to talk to you! That's rubbish!

As an adjunct to the exercises in the manual, I have used David Burns's book *Feeling Good: The New Mood Therapy* (1981) extensively with offenders, many of whom have included the entire book in their relapse prevention collections.

Negative thinking isn't just the province of sex offenders. Most of us know about negative thinking at some level: the way our interpretations of what happens affects our moods, and how we can get into a downward spiral in which we engage in illogical but nonetheless depressing self-talk. Therapists should buy Burns's book too!

Offenders who are negative thinkers often irrationally predict negative outcomes to their attempts to lead offense-free lives. Hence the manual includes exercise sheets relating to this, and the notion of positive fantasy about successful outcome is introduced (Manual, pp. 116-122). Again, these are exercises that can usefully be done on a regular basis.

Personal Relapse Prevention Manual, Phase 2, Section C: The Relapse Prevention Collection

Section C of Phase 2 in the manual (Manual, pp. 125-152) provides simple frameworks to enable the offender to make a relapse prevention collection based on all the work he has done in therapy. The offender is asked to identify a detailed overall plan, and then to make reminder cue cards linked to his keeping out of his cycle, breaking out of it if he has lapsed, and getting out of maximum-risk scenarios. The exercise titled "Dealing With Lapse Effectively by Picturing Success" (Manual, p. 148) asks the offender to imagine how good he will feel after coping well with an early-stage lapse.

In this section of the guide, ways of helping perpetrators individualize plans, and ways of checking them out and monitoring them are discussed. It includes completed exercises from Phase 2, Section C, which are not intended as model plans, but demonstrate individuality and addresses thoughts, feelings, senses, and behaviors. The "collections" described therein are offered as examples in the personal relapse prevention manual (Manual, pp. 143-145).

If a relapse prevention plan is to work effectively, it must be truly individual. A relapse prevention collection should include more than just written plans; it should be an individually created assortment of books, tapes, pictures, and other objects that have special meaning to the offender. As far as possible, the items in the collection should, in combination, relate to all the senses as well as to thoughts and feelings. In compiling the contents of the collection, what matters is what works for the individual. The words and phrases should be the offender's own, the metaphors and similes should be those that have meaning for him. For example, one offender knows that listening to music is a warning sign for him, whereas another uses music as a means of relaxation to help him move out of his cycle. Another offender uses a particular tune that reminds him of his resolve not to reoffend.

Sounds are strong psychic cues for some people; others are more powerfully affected by visual stimuli or by smells. People sometimes demonstrate this by talking in different terms—for example, "I see what you mean" or "I hear what you're saying." Some people appear to have clearer recognition of thoughts than of feelings; others are the opposite.

Offenders who were themselves sexually abused as children have different ways of using their experience in relapse prevention. For example, Sean knows that he is on the route to relapse if he starts fantasizing about his own abuse; Matthew, whose collection is described below, uses the memory of how happy he was before he was abused and how miserable he was afterward as something to think about briefly to help him ensure that he does not reoffend.

Metaphors can help too. Robert dreamt up the notion of a seesaw and a diving board! He put all the good things in his life onto the seesaw, which he set beneath the diving board. Then he imagined emotional and physical lapses or steps that he might go through to get to the top of the diving board. The higher he climbed the harder it would be to get down, but it would still be possible. If he reached the top and jumped off, that would represent reoffending, and the effect would be the loss of the things he valued as he hit the seesaw and knocked the things sky-high! Another man, Warren, liked this notion, but couldn't go with the metaphor of a seesaw and a diving board! He created a cliff top with a little boat underneath full of the things he cared about. Jumping off the cliff, he would capsize the boat.

Developing and Checking Out a Plan

Relapse prevention is an integral part of therapy, so the therapist and the offender should review the relapse prevention plan regularly as the offender develops it. This is not a piece of work to do the day before the offender leaves the program. An effective plan is one that is alive and under constant revision. In order to keep this task positive and interesting—not a boring ordeal—it is useful to vary formats to include audiotaping, videotaping, drawing, writing, interviews, and checklists. Instructions such as "Draw a picture of your relapse prevention plan and explain it to the group" or "Make a video in which you describe and then act out what you'd do and say in different circumstances" may provide better-quality information than having the offender complete the same monitoring form repeatedly. However, the elements of the plan need to be collected together in a format that can be shared with members of the offender's monitoring group. It is useful to start with a written and/or videotaped exercise that the offender can revise and make additions to over time. Questions to ask in assessing an offender's relapse prevention plan include the following.

Is it his own or the group's? Ensure that the relapse prevention plan is the offender's own and that it relates closely to his main routes to relapse, which have been identified during therapy.

Does he know his own risk factors? Ensure that the offender knows his own cues, in terms of thoughts, feelings, and behavior patterns that indicate the earliest stages of his routes to relapse. Check to see whether the offender has taken account of the physical context for the plan—that is, where he is likely to be living, with whom, and how those people might reasonably be expected to act.

Does he recognize buildup? Ensure that he knows an overpowering force won't just come along and take him over. In most cases, there's a buildup to feeling this way. For example, check out that he knows how he builds up to a high-risk mind state. Check out that he goes beyond just recognizing obviously problematic sexual fantasies and child-related behaviors as risk factors. For example, my cotherapist Alice Newman designed a monitoring device that asks offenders to complete statements such as "I will recognize that my risk of reoffending is increasing when my sexual fantasies start to include the following elements . . . "; "I will deal with this by . . . ." She uses similar sentence-completion exercises relating to such offense-associated behaviors as emotional abuse of adults and the overt recognition of "accidentally on purpose" behaviors.

Has he developed matching coping mechanisms? Check out that the offender has a good range of coping mechanisms that are likely to work for him. Do they involve actions as well as thoughts? The more action the better.

Is the plan practical? Check out carefully with the offender how he sees the plan working in practice. Relapse prevention plans that have not been reviewed by a therapist may be filled with self-delusion and may act as subtle routes to relapse. For example, an offender who uses memories of being abused himself as a deterrent to abusing may be fueling feelings of anger and desire for revenge if he is feeling low at the time. On the other hand, if he is able concurrently to hold on to positive feelings, then his plan may be effective.

Is it a road to ruin paved with good intentions? Be careful to ensure that the offender has clear plans for putting his good intentions into practice. For example, "I'll make sure I don't get depressed" is just a good intention. Ask how he will avoid becoming depressed, and what thoughts, feelings, and behavior patterns will indicate the onset of depression. Ask him to envision that these plans might fail, and ask him how he plans to break out of a low mood.

Has he internalized the plan? Make sure that the offender has the plan in his head, not just on paper. Although many people find it very helpful to write down their thoughts and ideas, and use the personal relapse prevention manual as a workbook to help them develop their relapse prevention plans, relapse prevention is not an academic exercise. It must be realistic, and it must work in practice. It must also be at the fingertips of the person for whom it's designed. When a therapist asks an offender what he will do in certain sets of circumstances, it is cause for concern if he has to go and get his manual before giving an answer. He needs to be able to think quickly about what he will do, and he needs to be able to answer follow-up questions about what he will do in the event of various other problems arising consequently.

Help the offender to internalize his relapse prevention plan so that his coping mechanisms become second nature. Make it standard practice to ask offenders, without prior warning, to imagine themselves at different points on their routes to relapse, and then ask them to identify coping mechanisms quickly. In a nonresidential group setting, therapists can do this at any point before, during, and after formal group. In a residential setting, there is more scope to replicate the unexpected by asking offenders about scenarios and the coping mechanisms they would apply in more informal settings, well away from formal group work, such as in the evenings and on weekends. Offenders who feel that such questioning is an imposition need to remind themselves that relapse prevention is a way of life. The better prepared they are, the more swiftly and effectively they will be able to take appropriate action to deal with potential difficulties.

Where possible, therapists should have the offender use role play to act out scenarios related to routes to relapse. Ensure that the scenarios are identified by the offender and are acted out as closely as possible to real life as it is for that individual.

Has he shared it? Ensure that the offender has shared his plan with his support/monitoring network in the presence of the therapist. During the intervention program, ask the offender to identify what other people might notice about his behaviors and moods that would signify the early stages of a route to relapse. Review this regularly with the network.

Is he practicing what he's preaching? Where possible, ensure that the offender begins practicing his plan in real life and reporting on it regularly, prior to leaving his therapy program. Residential and custodial programs need to pay particular attention to regularizing callback sessions and links with ongoing community-based therapy relapse prevention programs, to facilitate this process.

Is the plan being monitored? Meet regularly with the offender and his support network to check out how successful both the offender and members of the network believe the plan to be. In questioning offenders about their plans, it is important to look together not only for positives but for areas of concern too. Relapse prevention is not about trying to be perfect; it is about recognizing and overcoming problems as well as rewarding positive work. If a plan appears to be working perfectly, there is probably something wrong in the area of honesty. Most plans need amending and improving.

The offender's answers to detailed questions about his relapse prevention plan need to show clear thinking, insight into self, realistic ideas, and an ability to be flexible in changing circumstances. Unprompted demonstration of good practical application of assertiveness work and positive thinking techniques are also valuable, together with demonstrable use of the relapse prevention support and monitoring network. Above all, an offender needs a credible plan to lead a satisfying offense-free life. Without such a plan, the offender may know what he ought to do, but lack the motivation to do it. The following dialogue illustrates how a therapist-offender discussion of the offender's plan might go.

> *Therapist:* Colin, I know you're a good painter and much in demand to paint your friends' houses. You've told them about your offending and some want to keep the friendship. Your probation officer is going to visit them with you to make sure everyone takes special care to make sure you're never left alone with a child. But, despite all the planning, let's suppose it goes wrong one day. Imagine you're working in the house alone and it's during school hours, but one of the children has come home early. She lets herself in with her key and suddenly she's standing next to you. What will you do?
>
> *Colin:* Think: That's a child, a child. I'd say, "Can you go and stand over there? Something might fall," or anything else I can think of to move her away from me.
>
> *Therapist:* Suppose while she's standing next to you, you're feeling aroused and she doesn't look like she's going away. What will you do?
>
> *Colin:* Self-talk again. Think: "Look what you've done, all you've had to build from scratch. Just for a few minutes, touching and getting a sexual thrill, look what you're going to lose, look what it's going to do to you." Okay, it's thinking of me, not her, but look what I've got now and what I wouldn't have, no freedom, maybe prison.
>
> *Therapist:* So what would you picture?
>
> *Colin:* A prison like in *Midnight Express*, nothing of your own, no peace, no privacy, people after you, physical attacks.
>
> *Therapist:* How have you felt after offending in the past? Do you feel good or not?
>
> *Colin:* Sometimes, good and excited and still exhilarated, doing something, getting away with it and not getting caught. Other times guilty, but I self-talk my way out of it.
>
> *Therapist:* To stop you it has to be something dramatic, then, about consequences for you?
>
> *Colin:* Yes, but sometimes thinking about what I've gained and could lose works better.
>
> *Therapist:* Sitting here imagining a scenario where you're on your own with a child next to you, sure, thoughts like that might be quite useful, but if it was actually happening, the physical presence of the desired person can be much stronger, the feeling's much stronger. So what can you then do?
>
> *Colin:* Walk away, first spark of flutter in the heart, little jump, little kick that you feel inside, walk away. If I'm in the middle of painting and that's difficult, make an excuse to go to the bathroom, and think how to get out.

Perhaps then look at my watch and say, "Hell, I'm late, I've got to be somewhere else. I'll have to finish this next week"—and go.

Therapist: What happens when next week comes?

Colin: Tell the people I've only got half an hour to spare, so I'll come when he [the friend] can help me do it, tell him what happened—maybe tell my probation officer first. Lots of other things could have happened in a week, though. There's a million and one possible scenarios. You have to think and move on your feet, and if you're feeling dodgy get out.

Therapist: What can you change about your daily life to reduce the risks?

Colin: Well, some things you definitely can plan for, like when to go shopping. You don't go to town shopping on Saturdays, the kids are all around. The shopping malls are open until late at night. I've got basic steps relating to how I offend that I don't take now. For example, the worry is that you get to that point, the temptation's there, just a foot away from you and you don't walk away, can't or don't want to. If all these thoughts start coming back, the frightening point is will the urge overwhelm and knock all your relapse plan down. So you have to look around you all the time, see what's going on. If a child looks at you, look away—don't smile, that's a killer. I need to be aware all the time, like at the newsstand, walk the long way around to get to the magazines I want, don't go past the teenage section!

Therapist: This isn't something coming along suddenly and overpowering you. It only feels that way when you've taken a lot of steps toward reoffending.

Colin: Yes, it's related to what my thoughts have been the week before. Even more reason to be aware all the time.

Therapist: One thing I wonder how you're going to handle. You like the buzz of being a risk taker. How will you replace the buzz in your life?

Colin: I'll get myself a motorbike. It's exciting, and good exercise.

Therapist: Okay, so you've got your bike, and you're whizzing around on it. You're in a lonely place and you see a young boy on his own.

Colin: So?

Therapist: So?

Colin: Look at what I'll lose, think of the boy and how he'd feel.

Therapist: What will you do while doing the thinking?

Colin: Ride away fast.

Therapist: You seem clear about steps leading to reoffending in different situations, and you've got clear plans to fit different situations you haven't come across yet. That's good. I also think you need to go away and make more plans about how you'll replace the buzz in your life.

This discussion shows some of the strengths and weaknesses in Colin's relapse prevention plan (Manual, pp. 126-130). It is a very self-focused plan, and it might be more effective if it has more emphasis on victim empathy. However, self-interest is also a way of strengthening an offender's resolve not to offend. It may work for Colin, but it is dependent on his having the offense-free life he values. He has a good monitoring group, and he has told the group members what the signs might be that he has returned to a low mood state. Colin goes quickly from the thought to the offense, so his monitoring pattern will need to match that.

Frameworks for Relapse Prevention Plans

The exercise in Phase 2 of the manual titled "Relapse Prevention Plan" provides a very simple outline within which the offender has the scope to detail a highly individualized plan. The exercise is progressive and enables the offender to collect information about himself that indicates his most likely routes to relapse and most likely lapses on the way.

Having collected this detailed information, the offender should have a much improved understanding of his pattern. This self-knowledge enables him, with his therapist's help, to devise a relapse prevention plan tailored to make use of his personal strengths in combating his known weaknesses and tendencies to follow negative patterns.

The two examples that follow show how two very different men devised their own plans using the "Relapse Prevention Plan" exercise framework. If the therapist thinks it would be helpful, these example plans can be shared with offenders who have similar offending patterns, to help them devise their own plans.

Examples of Relapse Prevention Plans

Matthew

Matthew abused intrafamilial children. While Matthew was in therapy, his wife and children were engaged in parallel work. He and his wife also began having sessions together, and she was involved in discussions about the plan and how it might work in the future should family reconstruction be considered. Clearly, prior to any possible return of

Matthew to the family, a detailed alert list would need to be identified in addition to the relapse prevention plan.

Matthew's Relapse Prevention Plan

1. List below your thoughts, feelings, and behaviors that have been noticed, either by you or by those close to you, in the periods leading up to your offending.

Thoughts

> That I would be better off if it wasn't for . . .
> That my childhood wasn't that bad and I enjoyed it.
> That only children care about me.
> I can't help the way I am.
> That when I was abusing the children they enjoyed it; look how happy we were together.

Feelings

> Feeling that I have nothing to lose.
> Feeling trapped by things out of my control.
> Feeling alone and that only a child could fill the gap.
> Feeling a need for pleasure that can only come from masturbation.

Behavior

> Isolating myself from other people.
> Increased masturbation to illegal fantasy.
> Showing a particular child more attention than others.

2. What patterns are formed by the thoughts, feelings, and behaviors you have listed?

> I start to feel bored and fed up; this then changes to a sense of being trapped by things that I can't change and feeling lonely. I then isolate myself from other people and start to think that I would be better off if it wasn't for so-and-so or something, anything that I see as out of my control and I am not able to change. I would then feel that only a child could fill the gap and make me happy.
>
> I would then start to run flash fantasies of my childhood and children I have already abused, seeing how happy we were and how close we were, that they cared about me and I cared about them. I would then feel a need to masturbate to illegal fantasy. I

would say I can't help the way I am, I didn't choose to be an abuser. I would then masturbate while running images of all the children I know through my mind, and selecting one that I could abuse. I would then build a framework of how and when.

My need to masturbate would increase, and each time I would strengthen my plans and remove any risks there could be to me. I would start to show the child more attention than the other children. I would spend as much time as possible around the whole family but still isolating myself for parts of the day in order to masturbate, all the time making my thoughts and feelings stronger about what "we" are going to do and how the child will be afterward. Any doubts or feelings about it being wrong would be destroyed or the responsibility put onto someone else, not me.

3. What kinds of thoughts, feelings, and behaviors do you think would be likely warning signals that your risk of reoffending is increasing?

Masturbation to illegal fantasies.

Minimizing what I have done to children and saying that's in the past now.

The view I have of my childhood and the abuse.

Wanting to be on my own for long periods.

Spending time around children when I don't need to.

The programs I select to watch on TV (programs involving children).

Books I'm reading and their content.

Feeling that I'm not in control of my own life.

4. What do you think would be your most likely routes to reoffending?

Getting to know local people with children, especially single-parent families, and not telling them anything about my past.

Going back to live with my wife and our children, while they are still looking only at the good me.

5. What would be your most likely lapses on the road to reoffending, and how do you plan to deal with each of them?

Fantasy: Reduce the need to a level I can manage.

Contact with children through friends: I obviously can't prevent this happening, but I can reduce the risk that I am to the children.

Meeting children in quiet places: I can avoid this happening but also plan how to deal with it if it does happen.

Changing my view of my childhood back to "I liked it," etc.: I feel this would be caused by other things, so I need to strengthen now what it was really like during my childhood so that I can't dump it so easily. I also at the time need to look at why I need to do this, because the outcome is need to fantasize, so I can look at what's causing the need.

Isolating myself from other people: By not moving back home but living out of the area, I will be able to build a new social life and make friends, but always making sure that I'm not hiding from my past.

6. List six things for you to think, six things you can say, and six things you can do to deal with each type of lapse.

[Matthew coped with his own victim experiences by pretending to himself that he had consented to abuse and it hadn't harmed him. In therapy relating to his own experiences, he recalled being happy as a very young child before he was abused. He remembers feeling very unhappy as a 6-year-old after being abused. He uses this in his relapse prevention plan to challenge his thinking errors about children enjoying abuse. It is important that in using this plan he should not allow himself to dwell negatively on feelings related to being abused, as this may trigger him into feeling sorry for himself and act as a precursor to offending.]

THINK	SAY	DO
Lapse through fantasy		
1. About me as a 2-year-old.	I don't need this.	Listen to positive tape.
2. About adults.	Why am I feeling this way?	Move from where I am.
3. The feelings I would lose.		Do something positive, such as painting, cooking a meal, going out to see friends.
4. What else could I do?	Look at all I'm going to lose.	
5. How I felt as a 6-year-old.	Come on, do something now.	
6. About doing something positive.		Avoid fuel, such as newspapers, books, TV.

THINK	SAY	DO

Lapse by contact with children through friends

THINK	SAY	DO
1. About me as a 2-year-old.	Should I be here? It's time I left.	Keep contact minimal.
2. About me as a 6-year-old.		When I leave I don't take any images with me
3. About the feelings I would lose.		Leave in a positive way.
4. Why am I here?		Consider if this is a good friendship.
5. About doing something positive.		
6. Feelings about friends.		

Lapse through meeting children in quiet places

THINK	SAY	DO
1. About me as a 2-year-old.	Keep moving, Matthew.	Keep moving where I was going.
2. About me as a 6-year-old.	They're happy, let them stay that way.	Ignore them.
3. About how they feel now.	Go home a different way.	Don't go back that way.
4. Why am I here?		
5. About doing something positive.		
6. Feelings about friends.		

Lapse through changing my view of my childhood back to "I liked it" etc.

THINK	SAY	DO
1. About me as a 2-year-old.	I didn't like it.	Listen to positive tape.
2. About me as a 6-year-old.	Look how happy I was before.	Move from where I am.
3. About me as an adult.	I'm happy now.	Do something positive.
4. Feelings about friends.	Come on, do something.	Avoid fueling feelings.
5. About doing something positive.		Read letters to me as a child.

Lapse through isolating myself from other people

THINK	SAY	DO
1. Feelings about friends.	Come on, do something.	Get out, meet people.
2. About doing something positive.		Look at why I'm isolating myself.

7. List one thing for you to think, one thing you can say, and one thing you can do if you feel in immediate danger of reoffending.

Think of me as a child, how happy I was when I was 2 years old and how I felt when I was being abused.

Say to myself, "They're happy, they have all the feelings that I enjoy now, don't take them away from them or lose them again."

Do move away from the child, if possible to talk to someone that knows about me, or else get home and listen to the positive tape, then log what happens and the feelings for future use.

Part of Matthew's relapse prevention collection is his "positive tape," which includes the following:

- *Side A:* a favorite relaxation exercise with music
- *Side B:* Matthew's own thoughts, recorded by him, on (a) replacing his most frequent negative thoughts with positive ones, (b) telling his own children that they are free of being abused by him and can talk to people about being abused without fear of him, and (c) writing a letter to his 6-year-old self, saying he understands and cares for him, and that he too can be free of abuse; and a favorite piece of relaxing music that he came to know during a very positive phase of therapy

Matthew was previously a profoundly negative thinker whose favorite type of thinking errors involved telling himself he was useless and a failure, that everyone was against him and didn't care about him, and that things were either good or bad, with nothing in between. Thinking errors resulting in bad feelings were precursors to his offending.

Matthew's cycle worked as follows: pro-offending thinking → poor self-image → expects rejection → sees it even if it's not there → behaves in ways that get rejection → withdraws into fantasy about children (including distorted thinking about himself as a child wanting abuse) → legitimates abuse → masturbation fantasy increases, including further distorted thinking, overcoming inhibitions, thereby further legitimating abuse → planning → targeting → planning → grooming → planning → acting. Feelings of guilt occurred at times, and these reinforced Matthew's poor self-image and feelings of worthlessness, thereby feeding the cycle further.

On the first part of Side B of his positive tape, Matthew challenges his main thinking errors as follows:

I made this tape because I wanted to, and it's okay to share my feelings. Because of the good feelings I have felt and shared with other people, I can share my feelings and this is how I feel:

> I am important to lots of people; they care about me and they worry about me.
>
> It is okay to get things wrong; I can always try again. I don't have to win at everything; it can feel just as good to lose. I know I am not going to get hurt just because I lose.
>
> If I have something to say, it is all right to say it; I don't have to wait to be asked. What I have to say is important to me and to other people.
>
> I can achieve what I want; all I have to do is try. I couldn't paint until I tried, and I am really proud of my paintings.
>
> It is all right to trust people. I shared my feelings and yes, it was painful, but I wasn't alone, people were there for me to help me through it, and I felt so good afterward. My world didn't fall apart; in fact, it got better.
>
> It feels good to do something for someone else just because I care about them.
>
> Other people need their own space just as I do; it doesn't mean they don't want to be with me.
>
> It is all right to feel down as well; I can hold on to my good feelings while I feel down. I can keep both feelings at the same time.

In the next two parts of Side B of the tape, Matthew continues the process in a rather different way but still follows the same theme of positive thinking. These parts of the tape draw on a lot of work done during therapy and provide a distillation of thoughts that allow Matthew to see a positive way forward. He focuses on the survival of his children, with or without him, and with the help of people other than himself. He also focuses on his own "inner child" and emphasizes that he cares for the child he was before, during, and after that child was abused.

The tape ends with a piece of music that emphasizes quiet, positive feelings and gives Matthew a sense of being at peace with himself. It conjures up images that he associates with these feelings. These are all images that have no association with offending and are focused on looking outside the self—for example, at the sky and seascapes.

Matthew's Relapse Prevention Collection

Matthew has gathered a collection that he can access and use quickly whenever he feels the need. It contains items that he can use to suit different moods, feelings, thoughts, and scenarios. Matthew's collection includes the following:

- One thing he can think, one thing he can say, and one thing he can do (drawn from the exercise above)
- His positive tape (described above)
- A photograph of himself as a young child (a visible image of his inner child)
- His paintings
- His covert sensitization tape

Simon

Simon is a single man who abused children who attended the school where he taught. He has been abusing young boys for most of his adult life. He justified this to himself by telling himself that his own experience of being abused in a similar setting had not hurt him and therefore it would not hurt the children he abused. He always got to know the boys well before abusing them, and told himself they were his friends, not his victims. His motivation to abuse was complex, including feelings of anger, loneliness, and sexual attraction to boys.

Simon's Relapse Prevention Plan

1. List below your thoughts, feelings, and behaviors that have been noticed, either by you or by those close to you, in the periods leading up to your offending.

   Thoughts

   > He looks very much like me when I was his age, and his family background is almost the same.
   >
   > He has very little communication with his father, and he has to shoulder many of the household jobs that I was made to. He probably resents this too.
   >
   > He will like a break from all of that, like I did.

I enjoyed sex with a man when I was his age and I used to go to him. It'll be the same for him. He needs attention and will come to me if I give him enough of it, and am good and generous with him.

I will get involved with the family so that it will look perfectly natural and normal for him to be with me.

If he says anything, they'll never believe it, or they'll cover it up if I do enough for them.

I'll be really open about his being with me, so no one will ever suspect.

I am sexually aroused by him.

He is special to me and I can see in his eyes that he will want what I want.

He will love all the special treats, and he'll never tell on me.

I know people say it's wrong, but they don't understand.

This is the way I'm made; God understands and will make allowances.

After all, I'm giving of my utmost, and no one appreciates it.

I'm entitled to some comfort.

At least I'm not getting women pregnant.

I would never do this to a girl because it damages and upsets them. Boys really want it and like it, like I did.

I'm sure there are others like me.

This is my only weakness and I'm so good at everything else that if it is exposed, people will understand.

The harder I work, the more easily I will be forgiven.

I think it is good for me because I feel I love him, and I am sure he will love me too, and I can work all the better then.

I will be thinking of him and organizing my life around getting in contact and being close to him.

He will become a loyal and loving friend. That's what matters; the sex is only a minor part of the friendship.

I could do without the sex if I wanted to; it's because I love him so much that I'm aroused by him.

If only he hadn't come along this would never have happened.

How lucky I am that we met.

I've got away with it in the past, why should it go wrong now?

Feelings

Unappreciated

Unloved

Used

Empty

Sorry for myself: poor me

Angry

Lonely

Hungry for comfort

Aroused and comforted by the thought of a new child

Bored with life

Aroused feelings related to being abused as a child myself

Anger and jealousy that I feel disconnected from the adult world

Withdrawn and suspicious of adults and friends

Self-centered

Aroused by a feeling of fear and anticipation about abusing

Angry and guilty about the arousal—but "I want"

Behaviors

Focusing my life and my work around the victim and his family

Neglecting other families

Neglecting adults who offered friendship

Spending more and more time in my house alone—feeling sorry for myself

Being short-tempered (frustrated!)

Unapproachable, defensive, and protective of my privacy

Sulky and looking for attention

Always complaining of all that I had to do, lack of appreciation, aches and pains

Looking for people to feel sorry for me

Being sarcastic and cynical on the one hand, and nice and helpful on the other

Unable to say "No," and still complaining that I never had my own space

Masturbating to illegal fantasy

Targeting for fantasy and future abuse

Being distant and acting the professional

Being a know-it-all with friends

Giving the impression that I'm okay and don't need my friends—
   but maintaining control by letting them know they need me

Acting the Mr. Superior who has it all together

Getting more and more involved in work and projects

Having to have everything perfect and finished on time

Obsessed with being on time and having the house perfect

"Things" becoming far more important than usual; anything to
   take the focus away from me, and yet using all of it for disap-
   pointment, anger, and poor me

Never taking time out or a day off for recreation

Being critical of others for having leisure

2. What patterns are formed by the thoughts, feelings, and behaviors you
   have listed?

A very selfish pattern of poor me as the predominant color.

A bit like a Fair Isle sweater, where only the person who knitted it
   knows how it works. When to put in the Mr. Nice Guy, Mr. Superior,
   Mr. Unapproachable, or Mr. Angry, Mr. Workaholic, and Mr. No-
   body Loves Me.

A pattern with one goal: the targeting and abuse of a child, and
   where this becomes the focus on the pattern for the knitter but is
   used to distract others by their preoccupation with the multiplicity
   of color and design.

Being inconsistent, yet a stickler for him, being out of control, yet wanting to organize and control everybody. Being sociable, yet wallow-
   ing in self-pity and anger. Being secretive and devious, yet
   pretending to be open and hospitable. Dumping blame and guilt
   on others by being self-righteous and pompous.

A pattern with more and more time spent on the focus of wanting to
   abuse, and organizing everything and everybody around that focus, but being the only one with the information on where everything is leading.

3. What kinds of thoughts, feelings, and behaviors do you think would be
   likely warning signals that your risk of reoffending is increasing?

Thoughts

I can manage on my own.

I don't need support and control.

I'm okay now to be involved with children and their families. It
   would all be different from before.

I want to test the program.

It would be okay to have the odd target victim or the odd illegal fantasy; I'll never hands-on abuse again.

I really only want friendship with children; I'll be able to keep sex abuse out of it.

The legal age of consent is low in other countries; we just have a cultural problem here.

REALLY DANGEROUS THOUGHT: BOYS LIKE SEX WITH ADULTS. THE CHIMES OF BIG BEN WOULD BE RINGING HERE!

Feelings

Feeling I'm worthless

Feeling unable to make good what I've done wrong

Feeling lonely and distrustful of adult friends

Feeling isolated

Feeling angry and sexually aroused—feeling unable to deal properly with either

Feeling out of control

Feeling that nothing is going right

Feeling a need for comfort

Feeling a need to masturbate for comfort and release of angry feelings

Feeling comfortable in the presence of children; seeking them out to get that feeling

Feeling irresponsible; to hell with everyone and everything—blaming others for my feelings and making them responsible

Behaviors

THE MOST DANGEROUS: ISOLATING MYSELF FROM OTHER ADULTS AND ADULT RELATIONSHIPS

Acting independent and self-sufficient

Masturbating to illegal fantasy

Playing with fire by associating with and trying to get near children

Getting so involved in work or projects that I am not taking time to look at myself, and my thoughts, feelings, and behaviors

Avoiding anyone who might be a challenge or a help to me

Pretending that everything is fine and that I'm in control

Being secretive about my movements

Spending unnecessary and excessive time with children or adults and children together, e.g., with families

4. What do you think would be your most likely routes to reoffending?

[It is clear from the foregoing that the main routes identified by Simon are the "just testing" route and the "high-risk mood" route to relapse.]

Complacency and denial of my desire to abuse children; an "I am cured" mentality—"It will never happen again because I don't want it to."

Targeting and illegal fantasy

Telling myself that I am in enough control not to go any further with the abuse

Letting myself be close to children, and telling myself that I really do love them and would never harm them again: testing myself

Hooking into negative and "poor me" feelings and ignoring and minimizing the positive feelings

Giving up work on my sense of self and well-being, feelings of being worthwhile, and taking time for myself to grow and have healthy and happy adult relationships

Taking on a job that involves children, seeking out ways of being alone with a child

Blaming others for how I feel and ignoring my own responsibility for myself

Avoiding contact with people who know I am an abuser and creating a whole new circle of people who have no idea what I've done and am capable of doing as an abuser

Setting unrealistic targets and setting myself up for failure and a "to hell with it" mentality and feeling

Not dealing with my anger, or denying it when I feel it

Ignoring my own "survivor program" and reverting to the pattern of distorted thinking about my own abuse

Ignoring my own sexuality and denying needs and feelings for adults and adult sexual relationships; That they are about choice, and how, when, and where to deal with arousal and the feelings and choices of others

Being fearful and untrusting and avoiding hurt or rejection and turning to children as a comfortable, controlling abuse

5. What would be your most likely lapses on the road to reoffending, and how do you plan to deal with each of them?

[Generalized negative thinking provides Simon with the excuse to offend. He clearly needs to focus on challenging his own thinking, not just about sex offending, but about his perception of himself and about life in general.]

ANGER AND "POOR ME," MAKING OTHERS RESPONSIBLE FOR HOW I FEEL

Deal with by: Looking at my anger states, why and how best to deal with it.

ISOLATING MYSELF FROM OTHERS AND LOOKING FOR PITY AT THE SAME TIME—AGAIN TO FEED ANGER

Deal with by: Keeping in touch with the difference between, and the feelings in, good positive time for myself, e.g., reading, walking, listening to music, or just meditating and relaxation, versus the smoldering restless feelings of cutting off. . . .

Keeping lines of communication open and sharing feelings and checking out behaviors and thoughts with others.

I AM STRONG ENOUGH TO DO IT MYSELF.

Deal with by: Remembering this has never worked in the past, and I need to remind myself that it's okay to need and ask for help and to be able to accept someone being there for me in a challenging and constructive way; not feeding into "poor me."

LETTING GO OF THE POSITIVE FEELINGS AND HOPES FOR AN ABUSE-FREE FUTURE, AND GIVING UP AT THE LEAST SETBACK WHETHER IT BE A JOB OR A FRIENDSHIP

Deal with by: Taking each setback separately and looking at it in context with the other events and feelings in my life; not making a mountain out of a molehill just so I can feed on it.

Recognizing and accepting that people are not perfect, that there will be pain and hurt as well as joy and happiness. Looking at my expectations and seeing if they are realistic. It doesn't have to be black and white, all or nothing. It's better to live with flexibility.

TARGETING AND FANTASY: FOCUSING ON CHILDREN TO FEED MY AROUSAL AND MASTURBATORY FANTASY

Deal with by: Recognizing and accepting when I find myself sexual-izing children, reading sexual messages into their playfulness and innocence. Seeing them as children and remembering me when I was a child, and what I want for them and would have wanted for me. Using my fantasy aversion thoughts and audiotape.

HOOKING INTO MY OWN DISTORTED THINKING OR THAT OF OTHERS

Deal with by: Recalling the truth about myself and how I really felt about being abused. Thinking that children do not want it or like it, that there is emotional, spiritual, and physical damage: the wrecking of a life.

IN PRISON, TELLING MYSELF THAT BECAUSE I DON'T HAVE ACCESS TO CHILDREN, I CAN FANTASIZE AND MASTURBATE ALL I WANT; NO ONE NEED KNOW AND I CAN STOP WHEN I COME OUT

> Deal with by: If I am not building on what I have achieved, then I am on the freeway to abuse. Illegal fantasy and masturbation are continued abuse of past victims and a powerhouse for creating future victims.

6. List six things for you to think, six things you can say, and six things you can do to deal with each type of lapse.

ANGER AND POOR ME

> Think: About how I have dealt constructively with these feelings and how good that made me feel.

> Think: Make a choice to stay with this feeling and you know where it has led in the past—to abuse.

> Think: About how anger cuts everyone out and puts selfishness and comfort seeking at the top of the list.

> Think: "Poor me" is refusing to take responsibility for myself and focusing on blaming others.

> Think: I am okay to feel angry, but I need to look at why and where I am coming from in the anger.

> Think: I have a choice in this. How can I best deal with it in a positive and assertive way? Make a plan!

> Say: "I am not sitting on this rubbish."

> Say: "Get off your butt and talk to someone, especially if that someone is connected with the anger."

> Say: "Write down how you are feeling and where you think the feelings are coming from."

> Say: "Stop feeling sorry for yourself—ask yourself if it is your own fault and how you are using it."

> Say: "It is not the end of the world; you know better."

> Say: "I care about you, Simon, and this mood is not doing you much good—what will?"

> Do: Talk about the feelings and mood.

> Do: Stop blaming others or another, put myself in the frame.

> Do: Write out the scenario and the feelings before, during, and afterward.

Do: Accept responsibility for my own part and my own feelings and behavior.

Do: Be assertive rather than angry and deal with the scenario or person as soon as possible. Don't let anger build on anger and distortions.

Do: Mix with others and listen to them and let them in and not cut them off to feed the mood.

ISOLATING MYSELF FROM OTHERS

Think: I feel much better and more alive when I let others into my life and that positive beats the hell out of this crap.

Think: It's bloody cold, lonely, and isolated in this place and look where it leads me for comfort—to abuse.

Think: How I have used this to fuel the anger that leads to abuse.

Think: I am lovable and loving and depriving myself and others of the life that communication and sharing can bring.

Think: Now what are the masks and behavior I am using to achieve this and why am I doing it in the first place—what else is going on?

Think: Have I been targeting or already targeted for abuse, and am I just building up the anger and moods to excuse and justify abusing?

Say: "Get the hell out of here and talk about what is going on."

Say: "Simon, you are doing this to fuel anger, show anger indirectly instead of dealing with it—what the hell is going on?"

Say: "What are you hiding, what are you afraid of being seen—where's the secret?"

Say: "What are you not saying to another or others about your feelings about them?"

Say: "Where has 'poor me' ever taken you? You know where—admit you know how good it feels to keep out of this place."

Say: "Stop manipulating others and wearing the masks that dictate what they must say to feed the self-pity. Where's the life in it and where are you putting them?"

Do: Look carefully at *why* I am into this lapse or wanting to go into it.

Do: Talk or write to a friend or member of control group, or both, and say what is going on.

Do: Examine my use of time—is there time for me?

Do: Ask for help if work or confinement is getting too much for me.

Do: Check out the validity or truth of what I am blaming others for.

Do: Have a nice bath, dress up, and ask a friend out for the evening—don't go back to waiting to be asked.

AM STRONG ENOUGH TO DO IT MYSELF

Think: That's what you thought before and look where it got you.

Think: This is all about selfishness and control.

Think: Where has trust gone?

Think: Why do I want to get into this mode?

Think: This is just another form of cutting myself off from others.

Think: What's behind all this? What am I hiding?

Say: "Admit it to yourself—you know it is not possible to grow on your own."

Say: "Remember how things changed when you did let others be there for you."

Say: "Put down the mask of self-sufficiency and control, and take up the feeling of vulnerability and need."

Say: "Stop fooling yourself, you are not safe and children are not safe from you and the risk to them is too high."

Say: "Internal control is not sufficient—it's too vulnerable to life's experiences. External control and support are vital."

Do: Admit to any thoughts, and deal with them, that are leading up that garden path.

Do: Stay in contact with significant people who know my abusive disposition and can challenge me.

Do: Stop and deal with any fantasies that have a hint of dangerous independence.

Do: Recognize and accept my internal controls but don't make them exclusive.

Do: Keep asking for help when it is needed; don't claim "I can manage this on my own."

Do: Learn to delegate when it comes to jobs and work scenarios—others have talents and abilities too.

LETTING GO OF POSITIVE FEELINGS AND HOPES

Think: Why in God's name am I replacing good positive feelings with negative destructive ones?

Think: Where is this putting you in your cycle of offending?

Think: Where are these negatives coming from?

Think: Am I falling back into depending on my work for approval?

Think: Where is Simon in all of this? Recall your hopes and feelings, go through them one by one.

Think: How good it feels not to be abusing, not having secrets about abuse, and not killing the life and innocence in children.

Say: Repeat aloud, "I am of value, a loving and caring man."

Say: "I can do things for me, take time for me; then I can be of value to others."

Say: "Compare your life now and your feelings about yourself and others, especially children, with when you were offending."

Say: "Negatives lead to self-pity, poor me, anger, and offending."

Say: "I am loved, I know it, I feel it."

Say: "I *want* a better and better quality of life, and being positive is the only road."

Do: Get out pen and paper and write down the positives and the negatives.

Do: Deal with the negatives in a way that strengthens the positives.

Do: Examine the source of the negatives and why I am looking into them.

Do: Do something positive for myself or/and another, e.g., write a letter, make a phone call to someone I feel positive about.

Do: Do some physical exercise or play a game that involves others.

Do: Recall scenarios and people that inspire good positive feelings and bring in the realistic hopes for the future.

TARGETING AND FANTASY

Think: This is a child I am looking at.

Think: This child is entitled to a childhood, innocence, and freedom to be.

Think: What I have seen on the face of my victims and how they really reacted to me.

Think: I know now how I really feel about my own abuse.

Think: Stop sexualizing and examine my distortions and expose them for what they are.

Think: This is the fastest road to sexual abuse—get off it.

Say: "Look, see the child, look at the innocence and freedom, the sparkle and joy."

Say: "This child does not want sex with me, it is my wanting to abuse that is in operation."

Say: "Get your aversion tape running."

Say: "I don't need to abuse; life is taken away from that child if I abuse."

Say: "Call for help, seek distraction."

Say: "Call on all the other fantasies that give me life and excitement."

Do: Stop and examine my mood and behavior.

Do: Look at where I am in my cycle and take the steps to break it.

Do: Move away from the scenario and get involved in something worthwhile.

Do: Recall the work done in my program and why it was done.

Do: Put the child first and to be protected.

Do: Examine any distortions, expose them, and deal with them.

DISTORTED THINKING

Think: Why am I running these thoughts?

Think: What are these distortions minimizing or excusing?

Think: Am I feeding into other people's distortions to feel more comfortable about my abusing or being in prison?

Think: What is the real truth behind the distortion—what pain and growth am I avoiding?

Think: Am I using the distortion for a "poor me" state as an excuse to abuse or run an illegal fantasy?

Think: Remember how distortions played such a large part in my offending and my excusing my own abuse.

Say: "*STOP,* and expose the thinking for what it is."

Say: "Bring in the feelings and thoughts that put the distortions in their true light."

Say: "All my personal experience and evidence is in contradiction to the distortion."

Say: "Get into the truth—the reality."

Say: "What feeling is going with this distortion?"

Say: "Am I looking for excuses to go further into my cycle of abusing?"

Do: Get out pen and paper and expose the distortion in print.

Do: Write down the truth that challenges the distortion.

Do: Talk about what is going on with someone who can challenge the distortion and feed back reality.

Do: If talking is not possible, write.

Do: Read and study the real information about sexual abuse and its effects on children and adults.

Do: Remember the distortions that buried my own feelings about being abused and that ignore the feelings of my victims.

IN PRISON

[Simon came into therapy on a voluntary basis. While in his program, he admitted his offending to the police and consequently faced court and probable imprisonment. In prison, Simon could find plenty of excuses to sink back into feeling angry and sorry for himself; knowing the risks, he worked out a plan for holding onto what he had learned in therapy.]

Think: I do not cease to be an abuser because I am in prison.

Think: This can be a minefield for distortions.

Think: If I am not growing I am just going back to abuse.

Think: This is only a stage in my life; I can use it positively.

Think: I will have my ups and downs, but the downs do not have to lead me into illegal fantasy and masturbation for comfort.

Think: Remember that I am not alone, I have the strength of my friends and friendship and have a life to look forward to.

Say: "Time will pass, but I can use it constructively."

Say: "Take time to be positive about myself."

Say: "Keep in contact with my journey by being in touch with those who travel with me."

Say: "Missing friends does not mean negative lonely."

Say: "Recall the real positives of letting others be there for me and they are still there and with me."

Say: "This experience will strengthen my desire for an abuse-free life and make me more aware of the seriousness and evil of sexual abuse of children."

Do: Keep myself clean and tidy.

Do: Take pride in whatever work I find myself doing and do it well.

Do: Keep as much positive company as I can.

Do: Keep up my spiritual growth and sense of self-worth.

Do: See where I am as part of the process and look forward to moving on.

Do: Take it one day at a time and deal with issues as they crop up.

7. List one thing for you to think, one thing you can say, and one thing you can do if you feel in immediate danger of reoffending.

Think: This is a child I am wanting to abuse—a child, a child, a child.

Say: It's my lust, my sexualizing, my responsibility.

Do: Shout "help" in whatever way possible.

Simon's Relapse Prevention Collection

Like Matthew, Simon has put together a collection that distills key themes from his therapy experience. The items in his relapse prevention collection include the following:

- One thing to think, say, and do (as in 7 above)
- Favorite poems with an antiviolence theme
- Three books about people's ability to turn painful and negative experiences into something positive: stories of recovery and survival
- Chosen statements from his "Courage to Heal" workbook
- A copy of *Feeling Good*, by David Burns (a book about changing automatic negative thoughts into positive thoughts)
- A collection of items to remind him of the potential good quality of life
- A music tape
- Pictures of rainbows and oceans
- A relaxation tape

Building Effective Networks: Phase 2

In the Phase 2 material in the personal relapse prevention manual (Manual, pp, 143-147), the offender is encouraged to see members of his support/monitoring network as contributors to his relapse prevention collection.

As the offender moves through therapy, the number of people who join his planned external monitoring network may increase. The offender is asked to identify key people in his life with whom he could share his relapse prevention plan, and who could help him stick to it. In addition to those identified during Phase 1, these people might include the following:

- Named adult friend(s)
- Named adult family member(s) with authority
- Named adult(s) outside the family with authority
- Named adult(s) with authority within the local community (e.g., religious leader, doctor, teacher)

At this stage, in carefully selected cases, the nonabusing partner may take a more prominent role, providing the timing is right and the questions identified previously in the section "Building Networks: Phase 1" are being addressed. The nonabusing partner is likely to make a valuable contribution to the compilation of the alert list well prior to offender/child contact or family reconstruction.

Alert lists linked to the offender's cycle and his relapse prevention plan may help the partner to recognize signs of problems developing. However, if the partner has no one to discuss this with, she could easily be disempowered by the regrooming practices of an offender. Hence it is vitally important that the partner links closely with other members of the monitoring network.

Alert Lists

Alert lists should be individualized, with the warning signs identified by the offender himself, his partner, his children (where appropriate), and those monitoring or working with the offender. Where children are involved in identifying signals, it should be emphasized that they are not asked to do so with a view to their taking responsibility for monitoring the offender in the future. It is the responsibility of the offender not to offend, and of the nonabusing parent and other adults to pick up cues from the children and protect them appropriately.

The following are common warning signs that an offender may be moving toward or into his offending cycle. These are the kinds of signs that he and those living or working with him may wish to monitor. They will be relevant regardless of whether the offender returns to a family in which he has already offended or joins a new family. The alert list needs to be used as a positive tool, not as a trip wire.

Child-Focused Cues

- Tucking a child into bed without being asked
- Inappropriate touch, such as kissing on the lips, tickling

- Assuming the role of sex educator
- Inappropriate dress in the child's presence
- Buying non-age-appropriate clothing for the child
- Isolating a child
- Excessive interest in a child's social behavior or sexual development
- Favoritism toward a particular child
- Rigid authoritarian or unassertive patterns of discipline
- Undue interest in a child's hygiene
- Initiation of prolonged physical contact with a child

Partner-Focused Cues

- Shift in parental responsibility (either a shift in the perceived authority base or a shift in day-to-day patterns of responsibility)
- Unresolved conflicts; refusal to discuss problems
- Creation of situations that lead to rejection
- Aggression (verbal and/or physical or emotional)
- Increase in family isolation
- Poor privacy boundaries

General Behavior Cues

- Anxiety, depression
- Isolation
- Inability to complete tasks
- Alcohol abuse
- Loss of control over other behaviors (e.g., smoking, gambling, drug use)
- Negative change in sexual behavior pattern
- Use of pornography
- Sexual preoccupation
- Difficulty in accounting for time
- Overconfidence about not reoffending
- Failure to keep in touch with support/monitoring network
- Avoidance of appointments with professionals who are part of the network
- Involvement in youth work
- Work-related stress
- Rapid religious conversion, especially to fringe groups

■ Bedtime pattern that facilitates offending

Messages From Himself

Asking an offender who is moving toward the end of his program to engage in a videotaped discussion about what signs of slippage could be visible to different members of the monitoring group is a very useful way of developing an alert list and producing something that can act as a message to the offender from himself for use in callback sessions. The following dialogue illustrates this.

> *Therapist:* You've talked about a feeling of being cut off from other people as part of your lead-up to offending. What signs of that might your probation officers notice?
>
> *Paul:* I don't think they'd notice that easily, because I wouldn't be in that state in company.
>
> *Therapist:* Are there any ways they could tell you were headed toward that state?
>
> *Paul:* Yes. I'd be waffling, not being precise, not being honest about what I'm feeling, what's bugging me or what I'm pleased about, not being straight, drifting off.
>
> *Therapist:* Anything else?
>
> *Paul:* Not updating them on something I said I'd do. Not telling her what progress I'd made, or saying, "I tried it and it didn't work—I'll try something else." Not seeing things through properly.

Network Members

The production of a list of names by the offender is relatively useless if the named people are not vetted, interviewed, and given information by the offender's key therapist.

Vetting

Offenders may give the names of people who sound appropriate, but who may lack knowledge of sex offending patterns, or have collusive views which compound the thinking errors that the therapy program has been trying to challenge.

Those interviewing potential network members should ask questions which draw out the person's attitude to sexual abuse, to the offender's own sexual offending, to those he abused, and to the offender himself.

A Job Description?

When people have agreed in principle to be network members for a particular offender, it is important that the offender's therapist tells them exactly what the job will involve and describes how they will be supported by the offender's therapist and the network as a whole.

The network members need to be clear that their primary aim is to look out for factors that are known to be precursors to reoffending and to share them with other members of the network and, where appropriate, with the offender. Their role is not about taking responsibility for the offender's behavior.

Training

Network members may benefit from consciousness-raising training days on the nature of sexual abuse generally. Where appropriate, network members for a number of different offenders may come together for a training event.

Training should include the following information:

- Patterns of sex offending, including the cyclical nature of many patterns
- The four preconditions to offending identified by Finkelhor (1984): (a) the offender's motivation to offend, (b) the offender overcoming his own internal inhibitors (the relapse process), (c) the offender overcoming external inhibitors (the grooming and manipulation of those who may notice or take action to protect a potential victim), and (d) the offender overcoming the victim's resistance (grooming and manipulation, including threats, bribes, promises, and gratuitous violence as well as the imposition of distorted beliefs and values to gain compliance and prevent disclosure)
- Impact issues for victims on the receiving end
- Impact issues for families on the receiving end
- Routes to relapse, the relapse process, and relapse prevention

Sharing the Individual Relapse Prevention Plan

Both the therapist and the offender must recognize that lapses are likely. The most effective way of preventing relapse is for there to be an expectation that lapses, and plans for deaing with them effectively, will be discussed at regular monitoring sessions. In addition, there needs to be permission for offenders to telephone between sessions either to ask for help over lapses they are struggling with, or to share positive feelings about lapses that have been dealt with appropriately. An offender who is able to describe lapses and the way in which coping mechanisms have worked is far more ikely to be making real progress than one who denies that any lapses have occurred.

In particular, members of an offender's network should know the following about him:

- His patterns of apparently irrelevant decision making
- His common lapses
- His likely routes to relapse
- His high-risk scenarios
- All of his offense precursors

The offender should, with his therapist's agreement, select key completed exercises from the *Maintaining Change: A Personal Relapse Prevention Manual* to share with network members. Network members should also know about the offender's detailed plans for dealing with all of the above.

Support for and Sharing Between Members of the Network

Network members should be asked to report lapses or signs of offense precursors (e.g., mood changes in the offender) to the professional network member with statutory or key responsibility for supervising the offender. Where possible, they should repeat their observations in front of the offender.

Some network members may believe that it is enough for them to warn the offender, and some may feel that they want to protect him by not going to the network's key professional. Such members should be encouraged to recognize that external therapeutic help may be required, and that they are actually protecting and helping the offender most effectively by reporting him. If they do not report him and he does reoffend, he will be in danger of imprisonment and another victim will have suffered.

Where the offender's family members are involved in the network, they will need strong external support. It is emotionally very difficult for most people to report a partner or son, or brother, or father. It is even more difficult if they know that the person in question is capable of using violence against them or those close to them.

Where appropriate, network members should meet on a regular basis with the offender and the professional network member with key responsibility after the offender leaves his therapy program.

Phase 3

After Formal Therapy

This part of the therapist guide is linked to the Phase 3 material in *Maintaining Change: A Personal Relapse Prevention Manual* (pp. 153-162), which focuses on the need for offenders to engage in ongoing self-monitoring and to work with their external monitoring networks.

Phase 3 places emphasis on the need for post-intervention monitoring and callback and the need for the offender's long-term monitoring network to operate in a way that facilitates sharing of information. A key theme is that the network should be linked with someone who has the power to take action to protect children if this proves necessary.

In Phase 3, the therapist should encourage the offender to refer back to his Phase 1 work and to keep using and developing the exercises in Phase 2. Phase 3 has very few standardized exercises, because at this stage it is vital that any new ones should be tailored to suit the offender's individual needs and should be designed on an ongoing basis by the therapist and offender, as they review the relapse prevention plan together. What works for one offender may be counterproductive for another. Fine-tuning is essential.

Post-Intervention Monitoring and Callback

Perpetrators of sexual abuse appear to have greater difficulty in admitting to lapses than do other persons who indulge in addictive behaviors, such as drinkers, smokers, and gamblers. This is fairly easy to understand when one recognizes the possible consequences of admitting a lapse. A man who has abused his child and has been allowed back into his family may have enormous difficulty admitting a lapse, even to himself, if he fears that the consequence of admission is removal from the family, or even a return to custody.

Relapse in the case of perpetrators of sexual abuse is a reoffense against another person, and must be treated as such. This makes it even more important that the smallest lapses along the road to reoffending should be identified and dealt with appropriately. If the offender fears that his therapist will panic at the thought of his lapsing and would rather not hear about any lapses, he will not share this important information.

Both the therapist and the offender must recognize that lapses are likely. The most effective way of preventing relapse is for there to be an expectation that lapses and plans for dealing with them effectively will be discussed at regular monitoring sessions. In addition, there needs to be permission for offenders to telephone between sessions either to ask for help over lapses they are struggling with, or to share positive feelings about lapses that have been dealt with appropriately. An offender who is able to describe lapses and the way in which coping mechanisms have worked is far more likely to be making real progress than one who denies that any lapses have occurred.

Brian, who has been offense-free for several years, is able to describe clearly how he deals with lapses. The process he uses is a combination of self-questioning and incident analysis. This helps him deal with lapse positively and empower himself to prevent future lapses. He says, "When I notice a lapse I say to myself, 'Okay, this is a lapse. *Stop.* Now change your way.' Then I begin to work out the steps, which did occur but I did not notice." The following example from Brian's point of view shows how the process works:

Point 6: I recognized the lapse: I'm talking to a child. Having got out of the situation, I step back from it and look at Point 5.

Point 5: How did I get to be in a quiet place and "just happened" to meet a child?

Point 4: The reason I'm here alone is because I didn't ask anyone to join me for my walk.

Point 3: Why didn't I ask somebody? Because when I read the paper this morning there was an article about child abusers being put on registers and the community notified about where they live. I felt angry.

Point 2: Why did I read that article? I know reading that sort of thing creates negative thoughts. The reason I read it was because I feel bad about myself—that I'm a sex offender.

Point 1: Why did I feel bad about myself just then? Because a friend is getting married and I'm not invited to the wedding!

When I analyze all this, I see that I passed over the hurt of not being invited to the wedding without listening to my feelings and understanding that they were legitimate feelings. But then I must DO something positive about my void of loss. For example, on the day of the wedding, plan a day climbing, or something else that I'll enjoy. That way I can look forward to the day of the wedding even though I'm not going. Then I will not go into a negative mood and feed it with the steps that led to the risky scenario. When I look at it, the steps and the self-talk went like this: Steps 1 and 2, "You're not invited to the wedding because you're a sex offender!" Steps 3 and 4, "There is a register of pedophiles being compiled and you'll be on it." Step 5, "I must get away fast for a walk; isolate myself." Step 6, "Oh! Here's a nice boy on his own. I wonder what his name is!"

Brian uses this method of analysis regardless of whether he reaches a high-risk scenario. For example, he uses it to check out how he gets into high-risk mood states and to deal positively with the sources of any problems. Alongside this, he has what he calls his "pieces of gold dust" in his relapse prevention plan, and he monitors himself to check that these continue to form part of his offense-free life:

It must offer REAL LIFE—otherwise I'll eventually abandon it. I've gotten a thrill out of offending for many years. The illegal thrill must be replaced by LEGAL thrills that don't hurt people, and I've found those. It's important to RELAX when I'm tense, and I have good ways of doing that, too. I've made a host of ADULT RELATIONSHIPS with both men and women, so I don't isolate myself anymore and I've learned to listen to and be interested in other people.

Suggested Format for a Callback Session

Prior to a post-intervention callback session with an offender, the therapist should contact all those involved in the offender's monitoring network for feedback. The session itself might effectively run as described below.

New "Breaking the Cycle" Videotape

The offender makes a new 5- to 10-minute "breaking the cycle" videotape alone; in this tape, he tries to recall his relapse prevention plan, without referring to any written materials. He identifies what has worked well and what has been problematic, as well as any lapses and how he has dealt with them.

Interview. The offender and therapist watch the tape and discuss it. In addition to questions specific to the tape, the therapist asks:

- How do you think you're doing?
- What would those monitoring you say?
- What would family members say?
- What do you remember best from the program?
- What areas of work in the program affected you most? How? How have you used that since leaving?
- What do you remember of your relapse prevention plan?
- What have you stuck to?
- What have you changed? For the better? For the worse?
- What are the weaknesses in the plan?
- What are the strengths?
- How are you using your monitoring group? Are there times when you stop yourself from using the group? How do you do that?
- On a scale of 0 to 10, how satisfactory does life seem at present? Explain.
- On a scale of 0 to 10, how close to offending do you think you are? Explain.

Previously Made "Breaking the Cycle" Videotape

The offender and therapist watch the "breaking the cycle" videotape the offender made when he left the intervention program or, if he has been out of the program for a while, the one he made at the end of his last callback session. Seeing and hearing himself holding forth about his good intentions can be both salutary and empowering.

Interview. The discussion that follows might include questions such as the following:

- What did you forget?
- What messages from the you leaving the program would you most like to keep and use?
- If you forgot some key ones, why do you think that was?
- Under what circumstances are you most likely to forget them?
- Which routes to relapse have you started going down? Check them all out and include emotional and physical risk factors.

- If there was a risky mood-state route to relapse, describe the buildup to it.
- What seemingly irrelevant decisions have you made?
- Which emotional and physical risk factors feel closest to home for you?
- When do you feel motivated?
- When do you feel like giving up?
- When you feel like giving up, how do you make it other people's fault?
- Describe a typical day when you feel motivated toward an offense-free life.
- Describe a day when you've felt like giving up.
- How do you know when you're conning others? What do you/can you do to change that?
- How do you know when you're conning yourself? What do you/can you do to change that?

The therapist can usefully look for lifestyle issues, events, people, thoughts, feelings, the part played by self-talk, and the role of senses in what worked and what didn't. Look for interplay among all these factors.

Detailed Analysis of the Relapse Prevention Plan

If the offender has had difficulty remembering his relapse prevention plan, he and the therapist may decide to go through the plan in detail. Unworkable relapse prevention plans tend to be those that are full of good intentions without explicit planning for how to deal with difficult scenarios and how to realize the good intentions.

It is important that the therapist keep a copy of the relapse prevention plan, as an offender who is eager to relapse often "loses" his copy. This should be seen as a lapse in itself.

Analyzing Lapses

Where lapses are identified, the therapist asks questions such as the following:

- What did you do?
- What did you do before lapsing?
- What mood were you in before and during the lapse?

- What mood were you in after lapsing?
- How did you handle the lapse?
- What was the effect of the way you handled it?
- What mood were you in after that?
- Was this the first lapse, or did other lapses predate it?
- Which route to relapse do you think you were going down?
- How do you think you got there?
- What action can you take to avoid going into that particular route again?

The offender considers what he thinks he can realistically do differently and identifies one or two new ways of preventing lapse. Where the high-risk mood or mind-state route to relapse is indicated, this should involve something related to improving his lifestyle and his attitude toward it. He may need a refresher in "thinking positive." This problem and the related plan should be relayed by the therapist and the offender to other key people in the offender's network.

Questions the therapist asks might include the following:

- What plans will you make for the future, based on what works and what doesn't work?
- How can you strengthen your plan?
- How will you make sure you carry out your good intentions?
- What pictures, sounds, and smells will help you stick to your good intentions? How will you use those?
- How can you improve your relapse prevention collection to make it more dynamic?
- How can you make your offense-free life more attractive? How will you take its temperature?
- When it's going downhill, what will you do to pull it back up?
- Give an update on what you, and members of your monitoring network, are likely to notice about you before, during, and after lapses. What warning signals might there be? How will you deal with them?
- Even if people try to challenge you, you might not be listening. What would be the most effective way of getting you listening again?

Updating the "Breaking the Cycle" Videotape

The offender makes a videotape updating his relapse prevention plan and identifying courses of action discussed during the session, plus "Five Key Messages to My Monitoring Group" and "Five Messages From Myself to Myself."

New Work to Do

Exercises tailored to the individual needs and circumstances of the offender are set by the therapist and offender working together.

Sharing Information

Appropriate people are informed of the content and outcome of the session.

Callback Sessions, Weekly Groups, or Complete Weeks?

It is often difficult to assess behavior accurately in the context of a callback session. The therapist has to rely a great deal on the information provided by members of the monitoring network; hence good networking is of paramount importance. Ongoing monitoring of the relapse prevention plan in practice can be done in the context of a regular weekly group for people who have completed programs, but again, this allows insufficient time to focus on individuals, and if the group is a long-term one, there is the risk of it losing focus or even becoming collusive. My cotherapists Donald Findlater and Joe Sullivan have introduced the concept of callback weeks into our own residential program. This involves a group of approximately six men working together in residence for complete weeks at regular intervals. They are supervised by their therapists and work on an individual and group program specifically designed for them in liaison with their monitoring networks.

Continued Use of Phases 1 and 2 of the Manual

Some offenders may find that the combination of their reminder cue cards, lists of favorite exercises, and overall relapse prevention collections is generally sufficient to help them maintain an offense-free lifestyle. Others, however, may want to use the entire manual as a key part of their relapse prevention collections.

The way in which an offender uses the manual is a very individual matter. Some offenders focus on certain exercises or handouts in Phase 1 or 2 because these trigger their thoughts and feelings in antioffending ways. This can be related to logic, a feeling of enlightenment, or a positive memory associated with change.

Some offenders prefer to deal with lapse by following their own progress through therapy, needing to remember the distorted thinking of their early Phase 1 work in order to challenge it now, and then to remember the work they've done in Phase 2 in order to use it now. For example, one man for whom sexual fantasy about offending combined with high-risk moods was a major problem described how he uses Phases 1 and 2 post-intervention:

> I have found it more helpful to reread Phase 1 before Phase 2 when I am lapsing. The reason is that Phase 1 is more basic and therefore harder for me to ignore. Also, it contains a lot of distortions that I wrote at the time. When I read it they stand out like beacons for me to see. This in turn makes me think about what arguments I'm running, the things I'm saying to myself and how stupid some of it is. I've also started to underline parts of it that stand out, so they stand out even more now!
>
> Once I've read Phase 1, I can then go on to read Phase 2 in the right way. If I read Phase 2 first, it can act as a trigger for fantasy rather than helping me. The reason for this is I was pretty honest when I wrote Phase 2, the scenarios are real, so if I'm lapsing and I read a section about me being in a position to offend, I usually stop reading at that point and I'm all set to masturbate, so I really have to be careful what I read when!
>
> However, therapywise, Phase 2 is the better. It's much more hard-hitting than Phase 1, especially if you put the effort into it. Having to read Phase 1 before Phase 2 isn't a bad thing because it strengthens all that I've learned.

The same offender finds it particularly useful to keep his completed lapse sheets from Phase 2 in the back of his diary. He uses these to log any lapses and to prevent self-delusion. He added:

> I've started to fill them in during the lapse, which is even better. Because I work through the lapse I have a lot more information than I would have

·if I'd done it later. I feel good that I did something constructive and positive, and of course, it makes it harder for me to allow the next lapse to continue.

Self-awareness is crucial for offenders who have a high-risk mind-state route to relapse. One offender with such a pattern described how he wrote every night in his diary, putting down who he'd seen, how he felt, where he'd been, and so on. He looked back on the week's entries each week. He described what he found:

> It's quite interesting how different things seem. I can pick up a lot of thinking errors and other types of lapse this way. Some are obvious, others are not. I've noticed things like, I'm not job hunting, I'm isolating myself, I'm getting lazy, I'm laying in bed till dinner time, I'm not doing anything enjoyable or constructive. You notice it more if you look back over the week's entries than if you just fill it in and leave it.

The key to good ongoing use of the manual is collaboration between therapist and offender. Phase 3 is really a time for amending and fine-tuning exercises from Phase 2, and for creating new highly individualized ones that mean something special for that particular person and work for him in preventing relapse.

Working With a Network

One of the major difficulties of the network monitoring concept is not in putting together a network, but in making it work in practice. Open sharing of information among network members is vital. If a network is to be effective, its members need to take action to prevent development of some common problems:

- Professional jealousies and unhelpful scripts should be discouraged.
- Professionals should ensure that they are all concerned with child protection; they are not advocates for offenders.
- Therapists working with the children who have been abused should feel able to share information with the offender's therapist, and vice versa. This sharing of information should be between professionals, not necessarily with the offender. There should be confidentiality for victims, but nonconfidentiality for the offender.

- Representatives of law enforcement should have some level of involvement with the network.
- The network should have a structure in place to allow members to share any concerns about possible collusion with the offender by one of their number.
- All network members should be aware of the possibility of being groomed by the offender.
- The network members should use an "alert list" that is updated regularly.
- The network should tap into someone who has authority to take external action to control the offender or his environment.

Network members may find it useful to meet together and ask themselves the following questions on a regular basis:

- Who is ultimately accountable? Where does the buck stop?
- How do we know the relapse prevention plan is working?
- Do we really want to know? Are we inclined to panic at the slightest thing, or do we put on blinders? Or are we putting on blinders because we are afraid of panicking?
- What are we doing when we find out something that concerns us?
- How can we work together more effectively?
- When should we change the pattern of monitoring?
- Can we ever stop?

Conclusion: A Broader Perspective on Relapse Prevention

In order to be effective, relapse prevention programs must provide much more than knowledge of effective coping strategies. The offender must want to give up offending, and must have things in his life that matter more to him, and that he risks losing if he reoffends. For most offenders, the primary key to relapse prevention is the development of a rewarding offense-free lifestyle containing elements that motivate them to make use of the relapse prevention techniques they have learned. Even some habitual offenders are able to make this shift. However, many have built their lives around abusing others, struggle to develop the motivation to make real change, and may find the reality of an offense-free lifestyle very difficult indeed. Given this, we should perhaps be cautious about our expectations. Although some offenders will not reoffend, in high-risk, high-deviancy cases, we can only attempt to reduce the risk of reoffending. In some instances, reoffending is delayed; in others, the level of offending is reduced. Some men may reoffend, but the empathy they have developed and the coping mechanisms they have learned during intervention may work to allow them to reaffirm control and prevent further offending. This is not negative thinking—it is realism and recognizes the value of intervention. However, in the light of it, we should perhaps be even more cautious about making decisions that place offenders in close proximity to children they have abused already or might abuse in the future.

Many perpetrators of sexual abuse do need long-term external monitoring. However, as Marshall and Anderson (1996) ask, "How extensive does treatment have to be to keep recidivism rates at levels low enough to be acceptable, whatever they may be?" (p. 219). Marshall, Eccles, and Barbaree (1993) suggest that offenders might be stratified into risk categories and treated accordingly. In my view, although it may not be realistic to propose close monitoring of all offenders for the rest of their lives, priority should be given to three groups:

1. Those who have a long history of persistent offending and are at high risk of reoffending according to a risk-of-reconviction algorithm (Fisher & Thornton, 1993; Thornton & Travers, 1991)
2. Those whose offending is directly life threatening
3. Those who are likely to be living with vulnerable children

Priority for this third group may appear surprising, as it includes incest offenders, whose incidence of reconviction is generally low. However, the opportunity to manipulate and control in a family setting cannot be underestimated. If external monitoring is poor, and the perpetrator starts sliding into old patterns undetected, can we seriously expect children to tell a second time? The memory of what happened after the first disclosure is hardly likely to encourage them.

It should be possible to manage a low level of monitoring for all known perpetrators of sexual abuse. This could be done through national registers and authorities' sharing of information regarding the movement of offenders from one area to another.

We already have good-quality information about offenders who have attended intervention programs, but we are less good at using it. This could be done through the development of a database for the sharing of information about patterns and relapse prevention plans on an areawide, statewide, or, ideally, national basis. The database could be shared by law enforcement agencies, offender program delivering agencies, and the main child protection agencies, and could include information on all offenders who have engaged in programs, not just those who have done prison sentences—many offenders are never charged with their most serious crimes; they're caught on more minor offenses and are never sent to prison. The database could also include unconvicted abusers who have taken part in programs—agreement to be listed in the database could be made a condition of program attendance. The database could include the following details on each offender:

- Type of offender
- Previous convictions (and possibly alleged offenses)
- Target group
- Grooming tactics
- Risk factors
- Relapse prevention plan, including details of any external monitoring network

We also need to involve the community in offender monitoring in a way that empowers rather than panics people. Community notification without consciousness-raising about who offenders are and the relationship-based nature of much sex offending simply perpetuates the monster image portrayed in the media. Almost every offender is someone's relative, friend, neighbor, church minister, or youth leader, and no one, least of all the offender, recognizes him in the media image. Responsible public education can do much to create a safer, more aware society and reduce the risk of children being sexually abused.

Appendix A

Weaving Relapse Prevention Philosophy Into Intervention: A Sample Program

Sample Therapy Program

This sample program is based on my own experience in different contexts for intervention, and should be suitable for running in secure as well as community-based projects. It is aims led and provides a framework that can be used for running programs of differing intensity; hence it is adaptable for low-, medium-, and high-deviance offenders.

Assessment

Individual interview can be combined with psychological and psycho-physiological testing and group assessment work. The psychological tests used can inform intervention while acting as a benchmark against which to measure progress. The following battery of personality and offense-related measures used at the Wolvercote Residential Clinic, including the measures used by Beckett, Beech, Fisher, and Fordham (1994), can be used pre- and post-intervention.

Pre and Post Measures

- Offense-focused measures

Children and sex

Beckett, R. C. (1987). *Children and Sex Questionnaire: Cognitive distortions, emotional congruence.* Unpublished. (Available from Richard Beckett, Department of Forensic Psychology, Oxford Regional Forensic Service, Wallingford Clinic, Fairmile Hospital, Wallingford, Oxon. OX10 9HH, England. Description in Beckett, R. C., Beech, A., Fisher, D., & Fordham, A. S. [1994]. *Community-based treatment for sex offenders: An evaluation of seven treatment programmes.* London: Home Office Publications Unit. See pp. 155, 163.)

Sexual offense attitudes

Procter, E. (1994). *Sexual Offence Attitudes Questionnaire.* Unpublished. (Available from Oxfordshire Probation Service Research and Information Unit, 42 Park End St., Oxford OX1 1JN, England.)

Relapse prevention

Beckett, R. C., & Fisher, D. (1994). *Relapse Prevention Questionnaire.* Unpublished. (Description in Beckett, R. C., Beech, A., Fisher, D., & Fordham, A. S. [1994]. *Community-based treatment for sex offenders: An evaluation of seven treatment programmes.* London: Home Office Publications Unit. See p. 167.)

Beckett, R. C., Fisher, D., Mann, R. E., & Thornton, D. (1996). *Relapse Prevention Interview.* Unpublished. (Description in Mann, R. E. [1996, November]. *Measuring the effectiveness of relapse prevention intervention with sex offenders.* Paper presented at the 15th Annual Research and Treatment Conference of the Association for the Treatment of Sexual Abusers, Chicago; available from R. E. Mann, Programme Development Section, H.M. Prison Service, Abell House, John Islip St., London SW1P 4LH, England.)

Personal history

NOTA Database (1994). (Database of the National Association for the Development of Work With Sex Offenders. Available from Richard Beckett, Department of Forensic Psychology, Oxford Regional Forensic

Service, Wallingford Clinic, Fairmile Hospital, Wallingford, Oxon. OX10 9HH, England.)

- Measure of intelligence

Ammons, R. B., & Ammons, C. H. (1962). *Ammons Quick Test.* Missoula, MT: Psychological Test Specialists.

- Measures of self-image

Self-esteem

Thornton, D. (1994). *Self-Esteem Questionnaire.* Unpublished. (Available from David Thornton, Programme Development Section, H.M. Prison Service, Abell House, John Islip St., London SW1P 4LH, England. Description in Beckett, R. C., Beech, A., Fisher, D., & Fordham, A. S. [1994]. *Community-based treatment for sex offenders: An evaluation of seven treatment programmes.* London: Home Office Publications Unit. See p. 146.)

Personality

Blackburn, R. (1982). *Special Hospitals Assessment of Personality and Socialisation.* Unpublished, Ashworth Hospital, Liverpool.

Emotional loneliness

Russell, D., Peplau, L. A., & Cutrona, C. A. (1980). The Revised UCLA Loneliness Scale: Concurrent and discriminant validity evidence. *Journal of Personality and Social Psychology, 39,* 472-480.

Fear of negative evaluation

Watson, D., & Friend, R. (1969). Measurement of social-evaluative anxiety. *Journal of Consulting and Clinical Psychology, 33,* 4, 448-457.

Interpersonal problems

Horowitz, L. M., Rosenberg, S. E., Baer, B. A., Ureno, G., & Villasenor, V. S. (1988). Inventory of Personal Problems: Psychometric properties and clinical applications. *Journal of Consulting and Clinical Psychology, 56,* 885-892.

- Measures of victim empathy

Victim Empathy Scale

Beckett, R. C., & Fisher, D. (1994). *Victim Empathy Scale.* Unpublished. [Description in Beckett, R. C., Beech, A., Fisher, D., & Fordham, A. S. [1994]. *Community-based treatment for sex offenders: An evaluation of seven treatment programmes.* London: Home Office Publications Unit. See p. 136.]

Victim empathy vignettes

Hanson, R. K., & Scott, H. (1995). Assessing perspective taking among sexual offenders, non-sexual criminals and non-offenders. *Sexual Abuse: A Journal of Research and Treatment, 7,* 259-277.

- Measures of perspective taking

Interpersonal reactivity

Davis, M. H. (1988). A multidimensional approach to individual differences in empathy. In A. C. Salter, *Treating child sex offenders and their victims: A practical guide* (pp. 291-293). Newbury Park, CA: Sage. (Original work published in 1980)

Social desirability

Greenwald, H. J., & Satow, Y. (1970). A short social desirability scale. *Psychological Reports, 27,* 131-135.

Impulsivity

Eysenck, S. B. G., & Eysenck, H. J. (1978). Impulsiveness and venturesomeness: Their position in a dimensional system of personality description. *Psychological Reports, 43,* 1247-1255.

- Measures of sexual attitudes and arousal patterns

Multiphasic sex inventory

Nichols, H. R., & Molinder, I. (1984). *Multiphasic Sex Inventory manual.* Unpublished. [Available from H. R. Nichols and I. Molinder, 437 Bowes Dr., Tacoma, WA 98466-7047]

- Measures of self-control

Alcoholism screening

Selzer, M. L. (1971). The quest for a new diagnostic instrument. *American Journal of Psychiatry, 127*, 1653-1658.

Locus of control

Nowicki, S. N., Jr. (1976). *Adult Nowicki-Strickland Internal-External Locus of Control Scale.* Unpublished. (Available from S. N. Nowicki, Jr., Department of Psychology, Emory University, Atlanta, GA 30322)

Aggression

Buss, A. H., & Perry, M. (1992). The Aggression Questionnaire. *Journal of Personality and Social Psychology, 63*, 3, 452-459.

Caprara, G. V. (1986). Indicators of aggression: The Dissipation-Rumination Scale. *Personality and Individual Differences, 7*, 763-769.

Social Response Inventory

Keltner, A., Marshall, P. G., & Marshall, W. L. (1981). Measurement and correlation of assertiveness and social fear in a prison population. *Corrective and Social Psychiatry, 27*, 41-47.

Impulsivity

Eysenck, S. B. G., & Eysenck, H. J. (1978). Impulsiveness and venturesomeness: Their position in a dimensional system of personality description. *Psychological Reports, 43*, 1247-1255.

Measures and Exercises That Can Be
Used at Intervals Throughout the Program

Group environment

Moos, R. H. (1986). *Group Environment Scale manual* (2nd ed.). Palo Alto, CA: Consulting Psychologists Press.

Individual clinical ratings

Hogue, T. (1992). *Individual Clinical Rating Form.* Unpublished. (Available from T. Hogue, H.M. Prison Service, Abell House, John Islip St., London SW1P 4LH, England.)

Exercises

Eldridge, H. J. (1991). *Breaking the cycle: Offence description and matching relapse prevention plan*: Videotaped exercise. (Described in Part II of this guide, pp. 16-17, in the section headed "Monitoring the Offender's Progress.")

Eldridge, H. J., Findlater, D., & Wyre, R. (1991). *Offences, effects and who is to blame*: Videotaped exercise. Unpublished.

Motivating Offenders

Depending on individual need, this work may be undertaken prior to or in tandem with the early stages of the program. Common blocks and ways of overcoming them are noted in this guide in Part III, Phase 1, "Motivating Offenders: Working With Blocks to Receptivity (pp. 22-27, this guide)."

Monitoring Networks

Good practice for networking linked to a regular progress review system is described in Part III of this volume, in the "Building Networks" sections in Phases 1 and 2 (pp. 43-54, 101-107, this guide), and in the "Working With a Network" section in Phase 3 (pp. 117-118, this guide).

Preparation for the Main Program:
Detailed Analysis of the Offending Cycle

At this point, the offender is asked to complete exercises from Phase 1 of *Maintaining Change: A Personal Relapse Prevention Manual*. This provides homework to support individual and group work. An in-depth analysis of the offending cycle begins. Ideas for identifying the thinking, feeling, and senses cycles are described in this guide in Part III, Phase 1, "Working With Multidimensional Cycles of Sex Offending (pp. 27-43)."

To understand his cycle thoroughly, the offender will have to challenge his own thinking errors. Groups can be used very effectively to facilitate this process, and the therapist can set group members individual tasks to help them argue against their own distorted logic. The personal relapse prevention manual helps here, too.

In summary, each offender identifies the attitudes, beliefs, feelings, and behaviors that have led him toward offending as well as those that can help him resist the desire to offend. He relates these to his cycle, its active phases and phases of inhibition, and makes his first self-awareness and "breaking the cycle" videotapes. Provided the offender gains a real understanding of his own cycle at the beginning of therapy, he will be able to apply what he learns in future therapy to that cycle and the breaking of it. "Weaving" is about constantly making links between what is learned and relapse prevention.

The Main Program

Exercises from Phases 1 and 2 of the personal relapse prevention manual are set at intervals during the program. The therapist can give offenders whole sections en bloc or separate exercises, whichever integrates best with a given program and with the progress of individuals. Some men prefer having the freedom to use the entire manual in their own ways, whereas others are daunted by seeing all the exercises at once and feel pressured to complete them all quickly.

Most therapy programs include cognitive, behavioral, and psychotherapeutic components aimed at intervening in the offending process and breaking the cycle. Work can take place individually, in group, or a combination of both. Relapse prevention can form an integral part of either.

Individual Work

Although intervention often takes place on an individual basis, without accompanying group work, it is rare for the opposite arrangement to form part of good practice. Hence the sample group work program is backed by ongoing individual work (see Table A.1). Some work is done more effectively and appropriately in individual sessions, for example, behavioral work for sexual fantasy control, individually structured work on changing negative thinking patterns, and personal survivor and family-related work. This guide includes information on the last of these areas in the sections on building networks. The fine-tuning of an individualized relapse prevention plan is an appropriate task for individual work. Group discussion and review of the relapse prevention plan is invaluable, but if group is the only setting for such work, there is a danger that a "group plan" may be devised that is of little real value to each individual.

Table A.1   Sample Combined Individual/Group Work Program

Group work			
Core group work program	Additional groups (e.g., reasoning skills)[a]		
Individual work			
Sexual fantasy control	Restructuring of general thinking errors	Relapse prevention plan development[b]	Other issues
Family work			
Family work as appropriate, linked to offender's progress in the program and family members' progress in their own therapy; linked to networking aspects of relapse prevention where appropriate			

a. Participants in the program may attend additional groups at the discretion of their key therapists and those responsible for running such groups.
b. Increased emphasis on relapse prevention throughout the program.

Therapeutic Approaches

The program is primarily aims led, so although the specific exercises and techniques recommended have intrinsic value, in essence they are devices to achieve certain objectives, rather than ends in themselves.

A range of therapeutic approaches, techniques, exercises, and devices may be employed to achieve the desired objectives. These will vary depending on the needs of individual offenders and the repertoire of the therapists. Care should be taken to ensure that the approaches used are enabling, not humiliating, and that the instructions given are clear and well understood.

Cognitive approaches that stimulate offenders to use rational thought processes to challenge their own distorted thinking often constitute a useful starting point for therapy. Offenders may find this method less threatening than, for example, acting out offending scenarios in role play. As work progresses, more dramatic interactive approaches may be necessary to facilitate the development of real empathy rather than just intellectual awareness.

Group Work Program

The offender enters a core group work program that operates on a modular basis and has as a constant theme the offender's need to relate all that he learns to developing relapse prevention strategies suited to his own pattern of inhibitors and activators.

The modular program consists of four core elements, each of which is divided into modules that are different from but not necessarily more advanced than each other. This idea was originally conceived by Ray Wyre (Eldridge & Wyre, in press) for Gracewell Clinic's residential program and is used at Wolvercote Residential Clinic, in which setting each module includes ten sessions, each of three hours duration. However, the modular program can be adapted for less intensive programs (See sample program in Tables A.2 and A.3). In the sample program there are six sessions within each module, two of which focus specifically on relating new learning to relapse prevention. This program can be modified for closed or open groups to be run as a rolling or progressive program. At the end of each block of sessions, the offender completes a "breaking the cycle" video and another "self awareness" videotaped exercise. These are described in Part II of this guide, in the section headed "Monitoring the Offender's Progress" (pp. 15-20).

Offenders may attend other groups in addition, depending on their particular needs—for example, groups on improving reasoning ability and positive thinking or personal survivor groups.

Overall Aims of the Program

The overall aims of the program are to reduce the offender's risk of reoffending by doing the following:

- Challenging the offender's cognitive distortions, including generalized distortions, and those specific to offending scenarios

- Increasing the offender's empathy for his victims

- Increasing the offender's awareness of his pattern, with a view to interrupting it

- Increasing the offender's control over his sexuality

- Increasing the offender's ability to develop an offense-free lifestyle, in which he meets the emotional needs previously met by offending are met in other ways

Table A.2   Sample Group Work Program

	Module	Number of Sessions
"Breaking the cycle" video/self-awareness video		
Victim awareness/empathy	1	6
The role of sexual fantasy in offending	1	4
Sexuality and relationships	1	6
Assertiveness and anger management	1	6
"Breaking the cycle" video/self-awareness video		
Victim awareness/empathy	2	6
The role of sexual fantasy in offending	2	4
Sexuality and relationships	2	6
Assertiveness and anger management	2	6
"Breaking the cycle" video/self-awareness video		
Victim awareness/empathy	3	6
The role of sexual fantasy in offending	3	4
Sexuality and relationships	3	6
Assertiveness and anger management	3	6
"Breaking the cycle" video/self-awareness video		
Victim awareness/empathy	4	6
The role of sexual fantasy in offending	4	4
Sexuality and relationships	4	6
Assertiveness and anger management	4	6
"Breaking the cycle" video/self-awareness video		
Total length of modular program		
If one session is run per week: 88 weeks		
If two sessions are run per week: 44 weeks		

Table A.3   Typical Six-Session Module
(Example: Victim Awareness/Empathy)

Session 1	Victim awareness/empathy
Session 2	Victim awareness/empathy
Session 3	Victim awareness/empathy
Session 4	Victim awareness/empathy
Session 5	Relapse prevention ← victim awareness/empathy linked
Session 6	Relapse prevention ← victim awareness/empathy linked

Objectives for Participants

By the end of the program, each offender should be able to do the following:

- Challenge his own thinking errors

- Relate what he has learned in each module to his past offending

- Identify ways in which he can use new learning to break his cycle in the future

- Describe and act on a realistic relapse prevention plan that involves other people but does not rely on them

Arrangement and Length of Modules

Each of the modules within the four core elements may be run in blocks of varying length to suit the duration and intensity of the program. In the sample program shown, modules on victim awareness/ empathy, sexuality and relationships, and assertiveness/anger management are run in blocks of 6 weeks, with one session run each week. Wherever possible, however, sessions should be run at least twice weekly to ensure that all group members can participate fully and to increase the impact of the therapy. In our own residential program, sessions are run each weekday for 12 months. Where the only available option is to meet once a week, the size of the group should be kept to a small number, perhaps a maximum of five participants, to ensure the regular meaningful involvement of everyone in the group.

In the sample program, the module concerning the role of sexual fantasy in the offending cycle runs in blocks of 4 weeks, as additional individual work is done using behavioral techniques for sexual fantasy control.

Objectives for Each Module

In addition to the objectives outlined below, it may be helpful for each offender to identify his own set of objectives, related to relapse prevention, to be achieved by the end of each module.

Victim Awareness/Empathy Objectives

By the end of the program, the offender should be able to do the following:

- Recognize the impact of his whole offending cycle on his victims

- Describe how he controlled his victims and interpreted their behavior to legitimize his own

- Demonstrate empathy with victims of sexual abuse and his own past victims in particular

- Describe the ripple effect of his offending on others

- Identify how he will use victim empathy to avoid reoffending in the future, even if he is approached by a child who is acting out sexually

- Explain how he will use his greater understanding of victim issues to block arousal, pro-offending thinking, and targeting behaviors

The Role of Sexual Fantasy in the Offending Cycle Objectives

This module is used to complement behavioral techniques for fantasy control. By the end of the program, the offender should be able to do the following:

- Describe the part played by sexual fantasy in his cycle

- Describe how fantasy reinforces the desire to offend and acts as a rehearsal of offending

- Describe the distorted pro-offending thinking inherent in fantasy, and its desensitizing effect

- Use behavioral techniques to restructure his arousal to adult consenting behaviors

- Expect brief, "flitting" thoughts of illegal behavior and to learn effective ways of coping with such thoughts

- Recognize that masturbating to thoughts of sexual abuse is a lapse and describe ways of coping effectively with such lapses

- Relate what he has learned to his own offending pattern and to relapse prevention

Sexuality and Relationships Objectives

By the end of the program, the offender should be able to do the following:

- Identify the ways his attitudes toward sex and sexuality have helped him legitimize his offending

- Restructure his thinking patterns that objectify people, especially women and children

- Plan how he will use new thinking patterns about sex and sexuality to prevent a repetition of previous routes to relapse and to block thoughts that promote "I want, therefore I take"

- Demonstrate nonabusive attitudes toward sex and sexuality

- Understand the meanings of responsibility and intimacy in relationships

- Demonstrate knowledge of sex and sexuality in the context of positive consenting relationships

- Describe the differences between consent, compliance, and coercion

- Describe how he can use his greater understanding of these issues to change pro-offending thinking and behavior patterns and to replace abusive with nonabusive sexual relationships

- Relate what he has learned to his own offending pattern and to relapse prevention

Assertiveness Training and Anger Management Objectives

By the end of the program, the offender should be able to do the following:

- Identify whether anger plays a part in his cycle and, if so, the ways in which he has used anger to provide himself with excuses to offend

- Identify the links between lack of assertiveness (whether expressed through withdrawal or aggression) and his sex offending cycle, especially his excuses to offend

- Demonstrate appropriate anger management and assertiveness skills

- Demonstrate positive, realistic thinking patterns

- Identify scenarios in which he will use these skills as effective coping mechanisms to break out of old routes to reoffending

- Practice positive thinking and assertive behavior
- Relate what he has learned to his own offending pattern and to relapse prevention

Callback

A useful format for callback interviews is described in this guide in Phase III, "Post-Intervention Monitoring and Callback (pp. 109-115)."

Appendix B

The Relapse Prevention Questionnaire and Interview

The Relapse Prevention Questionnaire was originally developed for use in the Sex Offender Treatment Evaluation Project (Beckett, Beech, Fisher, & Fordham, 1994) as a research tool to measure to what extent individuals participating in treatment programs were aware of their risk factors and risk situations or scenarios and whether they had developed strategies to prevent reoffending. It is divided into questions that focus on awareness of risk factors and questions that focus on the use of appropriate strategies to avoid risky scenarios/situations, escape from them, or, if necessary, cope safely with them.

One of the authors, Dawn Fisher, comments, "In addition to being used as a research measure, the Relapse Prevention Questionnaire is of value clinically in that it can be used to gather information about individuals' awareness of their risk factors and situations and the strategies they have developed to avoid risk situations in the future and prevent reoffending."

Using the scoring guide enables a score to be derived for each individual, but it should be noted that the method of scoring is somewhat subjective, and the subscales are not statistically derived. Scorers should be trained in the use of the interview, and, where possible, interrater reliability checks should be carried out. The estimated level of risk simply reflects an individual's willingness to

AUTHOR'S NOTE: The Relapse Prevention Interview, developed by Beckett, Fisher, Mann, and Thornton (1996), appears in this appendix by permission of its authors.

admit to the possibility of future risk. It is not a score of actual level of risk.

The questionnaire has been adapted for use in the Lucy Faithfull Foundation's residential offender program, and has been further developed as an interview for use in the Sex Offender Treatment Programme running in prisons in England and Wales. Ruth Mann describes the interview in a paper she presented at the 1996 meeting of the Association for the Treatment of Sexual Abusers; she has commented that it is able to distinguish quite subtly between different areas of relapse knowledge and can inform on the effectiveness of a relapse prevention intervention. The version used in the prison program as an interview (Beckett, Fisher, Mann, & Thornton, 1996) is presented here.

RELAPSE PREVENTION INTERVIEW

by *Richard Beckett*
Dawn Fisher
Ruth Mann
David Thornton

Surname: _____

Forenames: _____

Date of Birth: _____

Interviewer: _____

Instructions to Interviewer

Introduce this interview with the following words:

From the work that has been done with people who commit sexual offenses, it is known that they go through several stages before an offense can happen. It will be easier for you to avoid offending in the future if you are aware of these stages, and the factors that put you at risk, and if you have worked out ways of controlling them. This interview is to see how good you are at doing that.

Think about the sexual offense(s) you have committed and then answer the following questions. Even if you do not believe you would be at risk of offending again, consider the factors that would be important if you were.

You may wish to allot a time limit for each answer to be produced.

1a. What feelings or moods would put you at risk of sexual offending again? Describe at least two different moods that would put you at risk.

_____

_____

_____

_____

1b. How will you cope with such feelings or moods in the future? Describe at least two ways of coping with them that you could use to reduce the risk of you reoffending.

_____

_____

_____

_____

2a. What thoughts, including sexual thoughts or fantasies, would put you at risk of sexual offending? Describe at least two different thoughts.

_____

_____

_____

_____

2b. How would you cope with such thoughts in the future? Describe at least two different ways of coping with such thoughts that you could use to reduce the risk of their leading to a sexual offense.

3a. What events might make you more likely to have feelings or thoughts that put you at risk of offending? Describe at least two different events.

3b. How would you cope with such events in the future? Describe at least two different ways of coping with each event that you could use to reduce the risk of their leading to a sexual offense.

4a. In what situations are you most likely to offend? What situations or places should you avoid? Describe at least two situations or places.

4b. How would you cope if you were in these situations or places in the future? Describe at least two different ways of coping that you could use to reduce the risk of each situation leading to a sexual offense.

_____

_____

_____

_____

5a. Many offenders go to considerable effort to set up a situation in which they can offend. How did you set up your offense situation(s)? Describe at least two different methods that you have used to set up a situation in which you could offend.

_____

_____

_____

_____

5b. What would be the warning signs for you that you were setting up another situation where you could offend? Describe at least two different warning signs.

_____

_____

_____

_____

6a. What sort of person would be most at risk from you? Describe this person in terms of looks, personality, age, attitudes, and so on.

_____

_____

_____

_____

6b. How would you cope if on meeting someone you began to have thoughts or ideas about offending? Describe at least two different ways of coping that you could use to reduce the risk of your committing a sexual offense.

_____

_____

_____

_____

7a. How might other people know you are at risk? Describe at least two different things that they might see or observe.

_____

_____

_____

_____

7b. What could you do to obtain help if you were at risk of offending again? Describe at least two different things you could do.

_____

_____

_____

_____

8. Who have you told fully about your past offending and enlisted to help you in preventing yourself from reoffending?

_____

_____

_____

_____

9a. Thinking about the excuses or justifications you used to give yourself permission to offend, describe at least two of them.

_____

_____

_____

_____

9b. How would you respond to such thoughts in the future? Describe at least two things you could say to yourself or do to stop this kind of thinking leading to sexual offending.

_____

_____

_____

_____

10a. Indicate on the following scale of 0 to 10 the likelihood of you committing a sexual offense in the future (0 is not likely at all; 10 is extremely likely). Circle the number that best describes you.

Not likely   0   1   2   3   4   5   6   7   8   9   10   Extremely likely

10b. Please explain why you have given yourself this rating.

_____

_____

_____

_____

_____

_____

_____

RELAPSE PREVENTION
INTERVIEW SCORING GUIDE

Basic Principles of Scoring

Each response is scored from 0 to 2 according to whether the offender's response meets certain conditions. It is obviously not possible for this scoring guide to account for all possible responses. Therefore, if in doubt, please decide which of the following best describes the offender's response:

0 = The offender refuses to recognize risk or the need to develop coping strategies. He shows no understanding of relapse prevention concepts whatsoever.

1 = The offender does not refuse to acknowledge risk and has some understanding of relapse prevention issues, but this is general or unsophisticated and could do with further development.

2 = The offender has a clear and appropriate understanding of his offending behavior, risk factors, and relapse prevention concepts and has developed well-thought-out, realistic, and workable coping strategies.

Q1a	SCORE	DESCRIPTION
	0	Identified no moods.
	1	Answered the question but with reference only to his past offending or gave an answer that is not a mood (e.g., "My mother"). Identified just one distinct mood. Include cases who use different words that describe basically the same emotion (e.g., "anger, rage, frustration").
	2	Identified more than one distinct emotion.

Q1b	SCORE	DESCRIPTION
	0	Identified no coping strategies. Include those who discount the possibility of the mood recurring or who say that "things are different now." Also score 0 for strategies that would put the offender at higher risk (e.g., "I would go for a walk along the canal").
	1	Identified only oversimplified or unconvincing strategies that are poorly thought-out, unlikely to happen, or unlikely to work (e.g., "I'll settle down and meet a nice girl"). Also only score 1 for offenders who mention only avoidance strategies (e.g., "I would keep away from children") or only escape strategies (e.g., "I would leave right away").

Q1b	SCORE	DESCRIPTION
	2	Identified more than one strategy that is well thought-out, realistic, and workable, at least one of which should be a cognitive strategy.

Q2a	SCORE	DESCRIPTION
	0	Identified no high-risk thoughts.
	1	Identified one distinct high-risk thought or gave as an answer a risk factor that is not a thought (e.g., "drunk"). Identified more than one thought but did not acknowledge the role of deviant sexual fantasy in his offending.
	2	Identified more than one distinct thought, including deviant sexual fantasy.

Q2b	SCORE	DESCRIPTION
	0	Identified no coping strategies. Include those who discount the possibility of the thought recurring or who say that "things are different now." Also score 0 for strategies that would put the offender at higher risk (e.g., "I would go for a walk along the canal").
	1	Identified only oversimplified or unconvincing strategies that are poorly thought-out, unlikely to happen, or unlikely to work (e.g., "I'll settle down and meet a nice girl"). Also only score 1 for offenders who mention only avoidance strategies (e.g., "I would keep away from children") or only escape strategies (e.g., "I would leave right away").
	2	Identified more than one strategy that is well thought-out, realistic, and workable, at least one of which should be a cognitive strategy.

Q3a	SCORE	DESCRIPTION
	0	Identified no events.
	1	Gave an answer that is a risk factor but not an event or that relates to his past behavior but not the future (e.g., "If a child is provocative—but this wouldn't affect me now"). Identified just one distinct event or type of event.
	2	Identified more than one distinct event or type of event.

Q3b	SCORE	DESCRIPTION
	0	Identified no coping strategies. Include those who discount the possibility of the event recurring or who say that "things are different now." Also score 0 for strategies that would put the offender at higher risk (e.g., "I would go for a walk along the canal").
	1	Identified only oversimplified or unconvincing strategies that are poorly thought-out, unlikely to happen, or unlikely to work (e.g., "I'll settle down and meet a nice girl"). Also only score 1 for offenders who mention only avoidance strategies (e.g., "I would keep away from children") or only escape strategies (e.g., "I would leave right away").
	2	Identified more than one strategy that is well thought-out, realistic, and workable, at least one of which should be a cognitive strategy.

Q4a	SCORE	DESCRIPTION
	0	Identified no high-risk situations.
	1	Gave an answer that is not a situation or that is not well defined (e.g., "stressful situations"). Identified just one distinct situation or type of situation (e.g., baby-sitting). (*Note:* Alcohol counts as a situation.)
	2	Identified more than one distinct situation or type of situation.

Q4b	SCORE	DESCRIPTION
	0	Identified no coping strategies. Include those who discount the possibility of the situation recurring or who say that "things are different now." Also score 0 for strategies that would put the offender at higher risk (e.g., "I would go for a walk along the canal").
	1	Identified only oversimplified or unconvincing strategies that are poorly thought-out, unlikely to happen, or unlikely to work (e.g., "I'll settle down and meet a nice girl"). Also only score 1 for offenders who mention only avoidance strategies (e.g., "I would keep away from children") or only escape strategies (e.g., "I would leave right away").
	2	Identified more than one strategy that is well thought-out, realistic, and workable, at least one of which should be a cognitive strategy.

Q5a	SCORE	DESCRIPTION
	0	Denied that the offense was set up in any way ("It just happened") or portrayed the offense as entirely opportunistic.
	1	Described one behavior that set up the offense situation.
	2	Described at least two separate behaviors that were used to set up the offense situation.

Q5b	SCORE	DESCRIPTION
	0	Denied that offending is planned or that it is likely to happen again.
	1	Identified only completely implausible, unrealistic, or overly inclusive warning signs (e.g., "being alone") or identified warning signs but denied the likelihood of their occurring or identified only one sign.
	2	Identified more than one warning sign.

Q6a	SCORE	DESCRIPTION
	0	Denied that any person is at risk or could not give any description.
	1	Gave a limited or vague description ("a woman") or a description that does not tie with his offending (e.g., offender against children claims adults are most at risk from him) or the description is reluctant and plays down risk (e.g., "Possibly women in their 20s, but basically I think I am safe with anyone now").
	2	Described at least one specific personal characteristic other than age or gender and in clear detail (e.g., "6- to 8-year-old girls with blonde hair and big eyes").

Q6b	SCORE	DESCRIPTION
	0	Identified no coping strategies. Include those who discount the possibility of the situation recurring or who say that "things are different now." Also score 0 for strategies that would put the offender at higher risk (e.g., "I would go for a walk along the canal").
	1	Identified only oversimplified or unconvincing strategies that are poorly thought-out, unlikely to happen, or unlikely to work (e.g., "I'll settle down and meet a nice girl"). Also only score 1 for offenders who mention only avoidance strategies (e.g., "I would keep away from children") or only escape strategies (e.g., "I would leave right away").
	2	Identified more than one strategy that is well thought-out, realistic, and workable, at least one of which is a cognitive strategy.

Q7a	SCORE	DESCRIPTION
	0	Denied any future risk or listed no signs.
	1	Did not deny risk but listed no signs or completely implausible signs (e.g., "I would tell the police") or denied that others would be able to see anything—only he would know.
	2	Listed one sign or more.

Q7b	SCORE	DESCRIPTION
	0	Had no ideas of ways to obtain help or denied any need for help.
	1	Identified an unspecified source of help only (e.g., "I'd talk to someone") or referred to people with whom he has not made contact (e.g., "I'd join a support group").
	2	Listed more than one specific source of help with which he has already established contact.

Q8	SCORE	DESCRIPTION
	0	Could not identify anyone to tell if worried or denied possibility of risk.
	1	Identified only one person or people with whom he has not established contact (e.g., "I would have found a group so I would tell them").
	2	Identified two or more people with whom he has established contact.

Q9a	SCORE	DESCRIPTION
	0	Identified no distortions or excuses or identified statements that are not distortions or excuses or that he does not understand as being such.
	1	Identified one or two distortions or excuses.
	2	Identified more than two distortions or excuses for offending.

Q9b	SCORE	DESCRIPTION
	0	Gave no strategy for responding to distortions *or* did not identify distortions.
	1	Described a vague strategy but without details on how he would put it into practice (e.g., "I'd get it out of my head"; "I'd talk to somebody") *or* described one sophisticated strategy only *or* described strategies that rely exclusively on others. Score 1 for a response of "Remind myself of the consequences" as a sole strategy.
	2	Described more than one sophisticated cognitive strategy, such as disputing the thought, reminding himself of the consequences of offending, using an aversive visual image, and repeating a phrase that will motivate him to avoid offending. Strategies are self-reliant and do not depend on others.

Q10a	Score is the number circled. In scoring the answer, it is important to make a distinction between seeing self at no risk (i.e., scoring 0) and seeing self at some risk (i.e., scoring 1-10). It is not possible to make judgments purely on the number given without taking the respondent's explanation into account. See his answer to Question 10b after his rating.

RELAPSE PREVENTION
INTERVIEW SCORING SHEET

Name: _____

Scorer: _____

Pre/Post-treatment: _____

Question	Score	Comments	Question	Score	Comments
1a			5b		
1b			6a		
2a			6b		
2b			7a		
3a			7b		
3b			8		
4a			9a		
4b			9b		
5a			10a		

Recognition of risk factors = 1a + 2a + 3a + 4a + 5b + 6a + 7a + 9a	
Identification of coping strategies = 1b + 2b + 3b + 4b + 6b + 7b + 8 + 9b	
Acknowledgment of planning = 5a	
Estimated level of risk = 10	

References

Abel, G. G. (1995). *The Abel Assessment*. Atlanta, GA: Abel Screening.

Abel, G. G., & Becker, J. V. (1987). Self-reported sex crimes of nonincarcerated paraphiliacs. *Journal of Interpersonal Violence, 2,* 3-25.

Abel, G. G., Becker, J. V., Cunningham-Rathner, J., Mittelman, M., & Rouleau, J. L. (1988). Multiple paraphilic diagnoses among sex offenders. *Bulletin of the American Academy of Psychiatry and the Law, 16,* 153-168.

Abel, G. G., Mittelman, M. S., & Becker, J. V. (1985). Sexual offenders: Results of assessment and recommendations for treatment. In M. H. Ben-Aron, S. J. Huckle, & C. D. Webster (Eds.), *Clinical criminology: The assessment and treatment of criminal behaviour* (pp. 191-205). Toronto: M&M Graphic.

Abel, G. G., & Rouleau, J. L. (1990). The nature and extent of sexual assault. In W. L. Marshall, D. R. Laws, & H. E. Barbaree (Eds), *Handbook of sexual assault: Issues, theories and treatment of the offender* (pp. 9-21). New York: Plenum.

Beck, A. T. (1976). *Cognitive therapy and the emotional disorders*. New York: International Universities Press.

Becker, J. V., & Coleman, E. M. (1988). Incest. In V. B. Van Hasselt, R. L. Morrison, A. S. Bellack, & M. Hersen (Eds.), *Handbook of family violence* (pp. 187-205). New York: Plenum.

Beckett, R. C. (1994). Cognitive-behavioural treatment of sex offenders. In T. Morrison, M. Erooga, & R. C. Beckett (Eds.), *Sexual offending against children: Assessment and treatment of male abusers* (pp. 80-101). London: Routledge.

Beckett, R. C., Beech, A., Fisher, D., & Fordham, A. S. (1994). *Community-based treatment for sex offenders: An evaluation of seven treatment programmes*. London: Home Office Publications Unit.

Beckett, R. C., Fisher, D., Mann, R. E., & Thornton, D. (1996). *Relapse prevention questionnaire and interview*. Unpublished manuscript.

Burns, D. D. (1981). *Feeling good: The new mood therapy*. New York: Signet.

Carey, C. H., & McGrath, R. J. (1989). Coping with urges and cravings. In D. R. Laws (Ed.), *Relapse prevention with sex offenders* (pp. 188-196). New York: Guilford.

Chaffin, M. (1996). *Working with unsupportive mothers in incest cases*. Paper presented at the 12th Annual Midwest Conference on Child Sexual Abuse and Incest, Madison, WI.

Cummings, C., Gordon, J. R., & Marlatt, G. A. (1980). Relapse: Strategies of prevention and prediction. In W. Miller (Ed.), *The addictive behaviours* (pp. 291-321). Oxford: Pergamon.

Eldridge, H. J. (1992). *Identifying and breaking patterns of adult male sex offending: Implications for assessment, intervention and maintenance*. Paper presented at the annual meeting of the National Association for the Development of Work With Sex Offenders, Dundee, Scotland.

Eldridge, H. J., & Still, J. (1995). Apology and forgiveness in the context of the cycles of adult male sex offenders who abuse children. In A. C. Salter, *Transforming trauma: A guide to aid survivors of child sexual abuse* (pp. 131-158). Thousand Oaks, CA: Sage.

Eldridge, H. J., & Wyre, R. (in press). The Faithfull Foundation's residential program for sexual offenders. In W. L. Marshall, S. M. Hudson, T. Ward, & Y. M. Fernandes (Eds.), *Sourcebook of treatment programs for sexual offenders*. New York: Plenum.

Faller, K. C. (1990). Sexual abuse by paternal caretakers: A comparison of abusers who are biological fathers in intact families, stepfathers and noncustodial fathers. In A. L. Horton, B. L. Johnson, L. M. Roundy, & D. Williams (Eds), *The incest perpetrator: A family member no one wants to treat* (pp. 65-73). Newbury Park, CA: Sage.

Field, L. H., & Williams, M. (1970). The hormonal treatment of sex offenders. *Medicine, Science and the Law, 10,* 27-34.

Finkelhor, D. (1984). *Child sexual abuse: New theory and research.* New York: Free Press.

Fisher, D., & Thornton, D. (1993). Assessing risk of re-offending in sexual offenders. *Journal of Mental Health, 2,* 105-117.

Hanson, K. R., Cox, B., & Woszcyna, C. (1991). *Sexuality, personality and attitude. Questionnaires for sexual offenders: A review.* Ottawa: Solicitor General, Canada.

Hogue, T. (1992). *Individual Clinical Rating Form.* Unpublished manuscript. (Available from T. Hogue, H.M. Prison Service, Abell House, John Islip St., London SW1P 4LH, England)

Jenkins, A. (1990). *Invitations to responsibility.* Adelaide: Dulwich Centre.

Laws, D. R. (1996). Relapse prevention or harm reduction. *Sexual Abuse: A Journal of Research and Treatment, 8,* 243-247.

Maletzky, B. M. (1991). *Treating the sexual offender.* Newbury Park, CA: Sage.

Mann, R. E. (1996, November). *Measuring the effectiveness of relapse prevention intervention with sex offenders.* Paper presented at the 15th Annual Research and Treatment Conference of the Association for the Treatment of Sexual Abusers, Chicago.

Marlatt, G. A. (1989a). Feeding the PIG: The problem of immediate gratification. In D. R. Laws (Ed.), *Relapse prevention with sex offenders* (pp. 56-62). New York: Guilford.

Marlatt, G. A. (1989b). How to handle the PIG. In D. R. Laws (Ed.), *Relapse prevention with sex offenders* (pp. 227-235). New York: Guilford.

Marlatt, G. A., & Gordon, J. R. (Eds.). (1985). *Relapse prevention.* New York: Guilford.

Marshall, W. L., & Anderson, D. (1996). An evaluation of the benefits of relapse prevention programs with sexual offenders. *Sexual Abuse: A Journal of Research and Treatment, 8,* 209-221.

Marshall, W. L., Eccles, A., & Barbaree, H. E. (1993). A three-tiered approach to the rehabilitation of incarcerated sex offenders. *Behavioral Sciences and the Law, 11,* 441-455.

Marshall, W. L., Jones, R., Ward, T., Johnston, P., & Barbaree, H. E. (1991). Treatment outcome with sex offenders. *Clinical Psychology Review, 11,* 465-485.

Miller, W. R., & Rollnick, S. (1991). *Motivational interviewing.* New York: Guilford.

Moos, R. H. (1986). *Group Environment Scale manual* (2nd ed.). Palo Alto, CA: Consulting Psychologists Press.

Ovaris, W. (1991). *After the nightmare: The treatment of non-offending mothers of sexually abused children.* Holmes Beach, FL: Learning Publications.

Perkins, D. (1995). Monitoring through psychophysiological assessment of patterns of deviant sexual interest. In H. J. Eldridge, *Maintaining change: A relapse prevention manual for adult male perpetrators of child sexual abuse.* Birmingham, England: Lucy Faithfull Foundation.

Pithers, W. D., Marques, J. K., Gibat, C. C., & Marlatt, G. A. (1983). Relapse prevention with sexual aggressors. In J. G. Greer & I. R. Stuart (Eds.), *The sexual aggressor* (pp. 214-239). New York: Van Nostrand Reinhold.

Pithers, W. D., Martin, G. R., & Cumming, G. F. (1989). Vermont Treatment Program for Sexual Aggressors. In D. R. Laws (Ed.), *Relapse prevention with sex offenders* (pp. 292-310). New York: Guilford.

Salter, A. C. (1988). *Treating child sex offenders and their victims: A practical guide.* Newbury Park, CA: Sage.

Salter, A. C. (1992). *Walking the walk, talking the talk: Indicators to effective intervention.* Paper presented at the annual meeting of the National Association for the Development of Work With Sex Offenders, Dundee, Scotland.

Salter, A. C. (1995). *Transforming trauma: A guide to aid survivors of sexual abuse.* Thousand Oaks, CA: Sage.

Sgroi, S. M., Porter, F. S., & Blick, L. C. (1982). Validation of child sexual abuse. In S. M. Sgroi (Ed.), *Handbook of clinical intervention in child sexual abuse* (pp. 39-79). Lexington, MA: Lexington.

Ward, T., Louden, K., Hudson, S., & Marshall, W. M. (1995). A descriptive model of the offense chain for child molesters. *Journal of Interpersonal Violence, 10,* 452-472.

Weinrott, M. R., & Saylor, M. (1991). Self-report of crimes committed by sex offenders. *Journal of Interpersonal Violence, 6,* 286-300.

Wolf, S. C. (1984). *A multifactor model of deviant sexuality.* Paper presented at the Third International Conference on Victimology, Lisbon.

Further Reading

Eldridge, H. J. (1991). Assessment and treatment of sex offenders. In G. Bradley & D. Lamplugh (Eds.), *The sentencing of sex offenders* (Report of an interdisciplinary conference) (pp. 61-65). London: Suzy Lamplugh Trust, in conjunction with the Criminal Bar Association.

Laws, D. R. (Ed.). (1989). *Relapse prevention with sex offenders.* New York: Guilford.

Marshall, W. L., Laws, D. R., & Barbaree, H. E. (Eds.). (1990). *Handbook of sexual assault: Issues, theories and treatment of the offender.* New York: Plenum.

McKay, M., Davis, M., & Fanning, P. (1981). *Thoughts and feelings: The art of cognitive stress intervention.* Oakland, CA: New Harbinger.

Multi-agency Working Group of Forensic Psychologists. (1994, July). Guidelines for PPG usage. *Forensic Update* (newsletter published by the Division of Criminological and Legal Psychology of the British Psychological Society).

Thornton, D., & Travers, R. (1991). A longitudinal study of the criminal behavior of convicted sexual offenders. In *Proceedings of the Prison Psychologists' Conference.* London: Her Majesty's Prison Service.

Wanigaratne, S., Wallace, W., Pullin, J., Keaney, F., & Farmer, R. (1990). *Relapse prevention for addictive behaviours.* Oxford: Blackwell Scientific.

Index

About the Author

Hilary Eldridge, B.A. (Honors), Dip. S.W., C.Q.S.W., is Clinical Director of the Lucy Faithfull Foundation, which works with adult and adolescent perpetrators of sex abuse, and runs an adult residential clinic for offenders providing intensive, long term therapy. The clinic also provides therapy for survivors and their families and trains professional groups in work with sexual abuse. Hilary Eldridge has specialized in work with sex offenders for more than 20 years. After completing postgraduate training at Leicester University, she worked as a probation officer and later co-founded the Gracewell Clinic, which ran the first residential program for adult sex offenders in Europe. She was Head of Training and Program Development for Gracewell. She has worked as consultant to a prison program and currently consults to community-based programs, in addition to directing the Lucy Faithfull Foundation's Wolvercote Residential Clinic. She has published book chapters and other materials relating to sexual abuse, including "Apology and Forgiveness in the Context of the Cycles of Adult Male Sex Offenders who Abuse Children" (with Jenny Still), which appeared in *Transforming Trauma*, by Anna Salter (1995); and "Barbara's Story," which appeared in *Female Sexual Abuse of Children*, edited by M. Elliott (1993). She is a member of the National Association for the Development of Work With Sex Offenders (also known as NOTA).

About the Contributors

Richard Beckett is a consultant forensic and clinical psychologist and Head of Oxford Forensic Psychology Service. He has held grants for research into adult and adolescent sex offending and is co-recipient of British government grants into the evaluation of community sex offender treatment programs and the treatment of sex offenders in prisons in England and Wales. He is an honorary research fellow at Birhimgham University.

Dawn Fisher is a consultant forensic and clinical psychologist working in a private secure hospital setting. She has worked in the forensic field since 1979, and has specialized in the assessment and treatment of adult and adolescent sex offenders. She is involved in a British government research project to evaluate the effectiveness of community and prison-based treatment programs for sex offenders.

Ruth Mann is a principal forensic psychologist who has worked with the Prison Service in England and Wales for ten years. She manages the Prison Service Sex Offender Treatment Programme, which runs in twenty five prisons, making it the largest scale program of its kind in the world.

Jenny Still, BA, qualified as a social worker in 1974. She has specialized in working with child abuse since 1977 as a practitioner, consultant, and teacher. As Senior Lecturer at the University of London, she set up and ran the government-sponsored national training program on child sexual abuse. She co-founded the Gracewell Clinic and is now Deputy Director of The Lucy Faithfull Foundation.

David Thornton, PhD, is a senior principal psychologist. He was responsible for introducing the Sex Offender Treatment Programme into prisons in England and Wales. He is Head of the Prison Service's Programme Development Section, which is responsible for the management of all accredited prison-based offending behavior programs, of which the Sex Offender Treatment Programme is one.